Alchemical Medicine
for the 21st Century

Spagyrics for Detox, Healing,
and Longevity

CLARE GOODRICK-CLARKE

Healing Arts Press
Rochester, Vermont • Toronto, Canada

Healing Arts Press
One Park Street
Rochester, Vermont 05767
www.HealingArtsPress.com

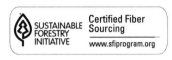

Text paper is SFI certified

Healing Arts Press is a division of Inner Traditions International

Note to the reader: This book is intended as an informational guide. The remedies, approaches, and techniques described herein are meant to supplement, and not to be a substitute for, professional medical care or treatment. They should not be used to treat a serious ailment without prior consultation with a qualified health care professional.

Library of Congress Cataloging-in-Publication Data

Goodrick-Clarke, Clare.
  Alchemical medicine for the 21st century : spagyrics for detox, healing, and longevity / Clare Goodrick-Clarke.
    p. cm.
  Summary: "Using the ancient art of spagyrics for treatment of today's health problems"— Provided by publisher.
  Includes bibliographical references and index.
  ISBN 978-1-59477-319-8
  1. Medicine, Magic, mystic, and spagiric. 2. Alchemy. 3. Homeopathy. 4. Detoxification (Health) 5. Longevity. I. Title.
  RZ999.G657 2010
  615.5'32—dc22

                                                                          2009054111

Printed and bound in the United States by Lake Book Manufacturing
The text paper is 100% SFI certified. The Sustainable Forestry Initiative® program promotes sustainable forest management.

10 9 8 7 6 5 4 3 2 1

Text design by Jon Desautels
Text layout by Priscilla Baker
This book was typeset in Garamond Premier Pro with Torino and Myriad Pro used as display typefaces

To send correspondence to the author of this book, mail a first-class letter to the author c/o Inner Traditions • Bear & Company, One Park Street, Rochester, VT 05767, and we will forward the communication.

For Nicholas, who first introduced me to Paracelsus and Samuel Hahnemann, and who has been my constant companion through many transmutations.

Acknowledgments

I record my debt to Manfred Junius, who was so generous with his knowledge, and to his alchemical partner, Siegfried Folz.

In memory of our alchemical laboratory work at Rožtěz in the Czech Republic under the instruction of Manfred Junius, I thank Michal Pober, founder of the Alchemical Museum in Kutná Hora; Brian Cotnoir for his humor, immense knowledge, and inspiration; Paul Carpenter, Art Kompolt, Steve Kalec, Guy Ogilvy, Mike Dickman, and all the other participants for friendship, wit, and wisdom.

Special thanks are due to Adam McLean, a pioneer who has done so much to facilitate the knowledge and understanding of alchemy.

Thank you to Ralph White, organizer of the New York Open Center Esoteric Quests in Europe. Each one has been a remarkable and transformational journey.

Disclaimer

I am not a medical doctor. I do not diagnose, heal, treat, or cure diseases. I recommend that people concerned about their health should see their medical practitioner for diagnosis and treatment, and follow appropriate advice. This book is intended for information purposes only and there can be no promises or guarantees about the results of using plant therapeutics.

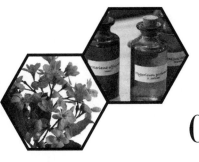

Contents

Introduction:
The Healing Art of Spagyric Medicine   1

PART ONE

Theoria: Alchemical Philosophy and Pioneers of Spagyrics

1 Alchemical Philosophy   8

2 Paracelsus   32

3 Paracelsian Philosophy and Spagyric Alchemy   47

4 The Vital Force: Samuel Hahnemann
and Homeopathy   60

5 Neo-Paracelsian Spagyrics   78

PART TWO

Praxis

6 Making Spagyric Essences   96

7 Plant Profiles and Therapeutics   108

Achillea millefolium   Yarrow   108

Calendula officinalis   Calendula   111

Carduus marianus   St. Mary's Thistle   115

Ceanothus americanus	Ceanothus	118
Chamomila	Chamomile	121
Crataegus oxyacanthoides	Hawthorn	125
Equisetum arvense	Horsetail	128
Foeniculum vulgare	Fennel	131
Galium asparine	Cleavers	134
Hypericum perforatum	St. John's Wort	137
Iris Versicolor	Iris	141
Melissa officinalis	Lemon Balm	144
Rosmarinus officinalis	Rosemary	147
Salvia officinalis	Sage	150
Sambucus nigra	Elderflower	153
Taraxacum officinale	Dandelion	157
Urtica dioica	Stinging Nettle	160

Notes	165
Bibliography	173
Resources	177
Index	178

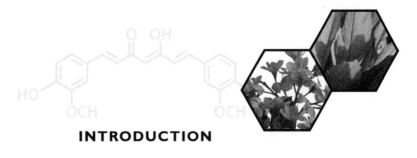

The Healing Art of Spagyric Medicine

It is curious that in this most advanced, affluent, highly educated era of human history, there is so much illness, much of it chronic and incurable. Often, orthodox medical intervention is not even directed toward the cure of the patient but only toward the life-long drug management of a condition (for example, asthma, diabetes, heart disease, and arthritis). The argument that we have more illness because we are living longer does not hold up; longevity does not necessarily result in disease—many people live very long lives in perfect health. We have more and better food, clean running water, and an understanding of hygiene unknown to our forebears, which should greatly increase our chances of achieving a long and healthy life. But unfortunately many spend years of their lives feeling not quite well, with no clear cause for their distress.

In 1900, there were three main causes of death: pneumonia or severe influenza, tuberculosis, and enteritis. All that has now changed. Since 1940, heart disease, stroke, and cancer have taken the place of these fatal diseases. Chronic ill-health and debilitating conditions are a huge cost to the happiness of human life. The National Center for Chronic Disease Prevention and Health Promotion describes chronic disease (heart problems, cancer, diabetes) as the leading cause of death and disability in the United States, accounting for 70 percent of all deaths.

1

One in 10, or 25 million people, in the United States have chronic disease.[1] There is general agreement that these diseases are preventable and that their incidence can be lowered dramatically by means of changes in diet and behavior, but this is seldom reflected in the way patients are treated for these conditions once they have manifested.

Pharmaceutical drugs are routinely prescribed to patients with the recommendation that they must stay on them for the rest of their lives, and yet underlying conditions and causes, whether physical or mental and emotional, are not addressed. Our conditioning leads us to see disease as something to be fought; the fight for health is a war in which the enemy (disease) must be eradicated, excised, or beaten. The means to this end often involve the pharmacological blocking of natural responses, surgical excision, and genetic modification. Most modern medical interventions fall into these categories. The medical paradigm is "to go against," for which we use the term *allopathy*.

Such an approach seldom leads to cure, and a growing number of people today do not wish to take pharmaceutical drugs, which burden the body with synthesized chemicals and suppress natural responses. Despite the billions of dollars spent on drug development, it is now widely recognized and reported that pharmacological use is itself a source of disease, with many thousands of people affected by iatrogenic illness every year.

Though modern Western pharmaceutical drugs tend to cause energy deficits, Ayurveda (the ancient medical system of India), Traditional Chinese Medicine, and most current alternative medicine systems (homeopathy, acupuncture, reflexology, crystal therapy, to name but a few) work to promote energy, recognizing that the balanced flow of energy through the systems of the body is one of the keynotes of health.

The World Health Organization (WHO) estimates that perhaps as much as 80 percent of the global population relies on long-established traditional medicine, most of which is herbal medicine. During the last twenty years of the last century, phytochemicals have been identified and analyzed as a new prospect for health maintenance. Bioactive substances in herbs and food plants have been found to play a significant role in protecting us from heart disease and strokes. Mainly, there has been a focus on food plants, but the range of investigation extends to a huge array of herbs around the world that have been regarded over centuries of tradition as healing agents. These plants contain biochemicals of highly specialized forms. Moreover, the complexity of phytochemicals in any one plant may have more significance than we thought previously. Some phytochemicals exist in plants in infinitesimal doses, but their synergy with each other in the same plant may be the important clue to long-term benefit. We stand at the threshold of a new era of medicine and at a point where it may be useful to engage with what has been known in the past about the importance of phytomedicines in all their various forms.

Energy comes from our food, of course, and from sunlight, good-quality sleep, and exercise, but also from phytotherapeutics. Plants contain nutrients and highly specialized volatile oils and resins in tiny amounts whose value in contributing to human health has not yet been fully understood. Like herbalism, *spagyrics* is a system of medicine based upon the energetic qualities of healing plants that contain substances that can help tune the human physiology and metabolism.

The word *spagyric* (German *spagyrik*) comes from two Greek verbs: *spao* (to separate) and *agyro* (to unite), in accordance with the alchemical maxim *solve et coagula, et habebis magisterium*—"dissolve and bind, and you will have the magistery." As the two Greek verbs suggest, the process of separating and combining implies a synthesis in which the finished whole is greater than the sum of its parts. *Spagyrics* has a long therapeutic history that can be traced back to the work of the great Swiss-Swabian physician, magus, and alchemist Paracelsus (1493–1541). Spagyrics refers to a branch of alchemy in which a therapeutic substance is separated into its constituent virtues, which are then recombined after purification. In plant alchemy the constituent virtues are essential oils, naturally occurring alcohols, and water-soluble salts (electrolytes).

Spagyric essences can be effective treatments for many ailments.

They are harmonizing and balancing. Further, when prepared properly, spagyric medicines are safe to use over a long period of time, and thus can relieve many chronic complaints. They are also invaluable when a person feels unwell but tests show nothing abnormal. At this early stage, before illness has become morbid pathology, the strengthening, balancing, and harmonizing effects of spagyric essences can prove restorative.

The *spagyric method* is the first level of practical alchemy and a way of enhancing the healing virtues of plants.

Plant minerals and oils act as catalysts to stimulate the body's own natural powers of healing and homeostasis. By stimulating faster and more efficient cellular activity, energetic plant essences help to restore the organs' capacity for self-regeneration. Spagyrics is an alchemical process that enables the capture of the essential minerals and salts in plants, purifies them (by ridding them of heavy metals), and then enhances their vibrational qualities. The result is a fine medicinal tincture, pleasant and easy to take, that regulates the systems of the body and is powerfully restorative. These tinctures are prescribed according to *homeopathic* (meaning "similar suffering") principles. The homeopathic paradigm has a long history going back to Hippocrates in ancient Greece. It has also been an operative principle of Ayurveda for centuries. Working with plants in this way will give you an understanding of practical alchemical philosophy and an insight into the profound healing capability latent in the vegetable kingdom.

But how is it determined that someone is indeed in need of treatment for a condition? Lack of energy is one of the first symptoms that all is not well. The subjective feeling of dis-ease, fatigue, apathy, irritability, or despondency may precede actual pathological change by weeks, months, or even years. These feelings are often indications that the body's resistance to external influences, stress, or viruses is diminishing. Energy deficit ultimately leads to local or systemic dysfunction, such as chronic fatigue syndrome; cancer; circulatory insufficiency; or chronic debilitating conditions such as diabetes, myalgias, and rheumatism. All chronic and recurrent infections may be traced to energy deficit.

Moreover, the rapid rise of diseases that are now partly or wholly resistant to antibiotics means that it is becoming urgent to seek out other forms of treatment. Those people who choose a lifestyle and medical system that build immune competence will always be the winners in the long run. They opt for treatments and lifestyles that promote energy in the body, including systems of health that recognize the need to build up energy in the body, so that the body is then able to cope with stress, fend off infection, and clear itself of toxicity. The means to this are dynamic medicines that stimulate a healing response in the body.

For a number of minor ailments, there is still a place for simple medicines that can be prepared easily and economically at home from herbs and common garden plants. Many people do this as a matter of course. Finding a few sage leaves, steeping them in hot water, and drinking the resulting tea soothes a sore throat, or drinking mint tea alleviates mild indigestion. This book is for those who would like to go further and explore the wonderful range of healing that is ours for the taking as soon as we step out into the natural, wild world.

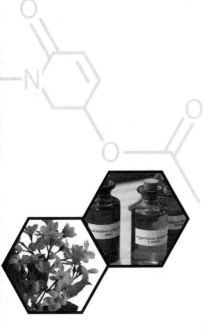

PART ONE

Theoria

Alchemical Philosophy
and
Pioneers of Spagyrics

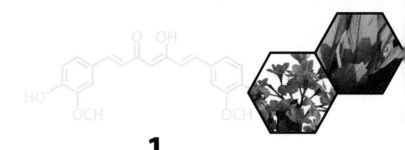

1

Alchemical Philosophy

Plants as Healers

Phytotherapeutics was once virtually the only form of medicine. Despite the continued and widespread use of herbs across the world and the fact that in the nineteenth and early twentieth centuries, herbal medicines constituted a high proportion of prescribed medicines in the United States, they are now usually categorized as *alternative medicines—* despite the fact that much modern medicine (including morphine, digitalis, quinine, and aspirin) were originally derived from plants. Many of these are now made from a synthesized form of the "active ingredient," which the pharmaceutical company believes it has identified and isolated. Today, the pharmacist in a white coat dispensing drugs in blister packs is far removed from the ardent potency of plants.

The medical science to which the modern world is now so subservient depends upon machines for assessing health and on technological interventions to correct ill health. The vital body is forgotten, as though the body were itself a machine, an assembly of parts. When something goes wrong, the diseased part must be located and "fixed." When each part of the body is seen in isolation, the long-term impact of emotional shock on the physical body as a whole is often discounted. Although some of our most highly respected modern drugs, such as aspirin, were derived originally from plant sources, herbalism itself is often disparaged because, it is argued, the active ingredient in plants is variable and uncertain. Yet the scientific search for the active ingredient is a sterile pursuit, because it rejects the integrity of the plant and its natural synergistic qualities. The active, vital principles of plants are complex and subtle, and the life force, chi, or prana of fresh, green herbs is contained in the sum of its parts—not in the isolated ingredient. In fact, the wonderful advantage of all phytotherapy is the synergistic effect of using the whole plant. For example, *Taraxacum* (dandelion), which is an excellent remedy for ailments of the liver, contains a high proportion of potassium, meaning that it is safe as a diuretic. The more we work with plants, the more we realize that nature brings the healing spectrum to us in neat, well-thought-out packages congruent with the needs of the human body. We now recognize that some plants contain compounds present in such minute concentrations that they are often hardly detectable by standard techniques, and yet they may be potent pharmacological agents.

Plants belong to time and the cosmos in a way that is unique in the vegetable world. Nourishment for plant growth may come from earth, air, and water, but the energy for their growth comes from the sun, moon, and stars. Whereas humankind and much of the animal kingdom seeks shelter at night, plants lie directly under the night sky so that their life rhythms are also mysteriously connected to cosmic time. Daytime is solar, as is the yearly cycle, and monthly cycles are lunar. The moon controls the rising and falling of the tide, the quantity of rainfall, and the rising and falling levels of water and sap. Earth-rooted plants reach ever upward, mirroring the aspiration of ascent and the marriage of earth and sky.

Waxing and waning through each month, the moon mirrors the light from the sun at various angles. At the time of the full moon, the moon is opposite the sun and is in synchronicity with it: as the sun sets, the moon rises. These continually changing angles of the sun and moon bring about electrical and magnetic changes in the upper atmosphere to which plants are subtly attuned. Flowers are recipients of light, and some plants are particularly oriented to the sun. The flowers of the genus *Helianthus,* such as the sunflower, follow the path of the sun: as the sun moves from east to west each day, so the flowers turn their open faces to gratefully receive the maximum benison of sunlight, which is stored in their great treasure hoard of a seed head. Light becomes matter and richly nourishing food.

How good it is to walk in nature, striding in wild places where the breeze is invigorating, the water is clean and pure, and the plants are vibrant and colorful. A healthy, natural countryside is not only green, but also should be full of bright flowers: clovers—purple and white; tall, yellow agrimony and mullein; charming wild orchids; and dazzling poppies. When we are close to Nature, the feeling that Nature is herself a living being full of wondrous powers is inescapable. Radiant flowers reveal to us her shining intelligence, full of the light of wisdom and healing power. In those moments, we ourselves may feel the benefit of nature's restorative energies, surprising ourselves by walking with a straighter back and a certain loose limberness that give each of our steps a kind of buoyancy and springiness that is all the more welcome for being unaccustomed. This is the healing presence that we capture in medicinal plants, many of which are the outcasts of the plant world, the misfit "weeds" that the fastidious gardener often ignores. Dandelion and goldenrod, plantain, teasle, and nettles—all of these are full of nature's healing virtues and can offer support for the ailing, even in quite severe illness.

A connection to the earth and to medicinal plants is our natural birthright. Animals have recourse to herbs, seeking out by instinct the grasses and weeds they need. This was also the human relationship to plants for long centuries of our existence. When we begin to work with plants, this connection to the original source of vitality and health is restored. You will find that plants come to you as healers and teachers. If you watch your garden through the seasons, you will find that certain plants seed themselves—and very often, they may be just the thing you need to assuage a condition. I have been amazed at how often *Hypericum perforatum* (St. John's wort) invades the gardens of the chronically depressed, and how rapidly nettles proliferate in the gardens of women of a certain age, and how hawthorn creeps unbidden into the gardens of the weak of heart. Among traditional herbalists, plants are valued as allies and collaborators in the field of health; knowledge of well-being comes from the plants, which offer themselves for healing.

Plants as Helpers

It is true, of course, that medicinal herbs cannot be regarded as completely safe: they contain many naturally occurring chemicals, and some contain powerful alkaloids. Their uncontrolled or ill-informed use is rightly discouraged. Yet the spagyric method of preparing plants does render them more vital and relatively safe. Any therapeutic agent can be harmful, and we should take great care in handling, preparing, and taking herbs. It is particularly important to be wary of taking herbs while also taking prescribed pharmaceutical drugs. The interaction of drugs and herbs is wholly underresearched. It is also clearly unwise to discontinue your prescribed medication in order to try herbal preparations. Always take due regard for your health and consult with qualified health professionals for the diagnosis and treatment that may be necessary for you.

Living among therapeutic plants involves a reassessment of value. Nettles, plantains, or chickweed are not usually tolerated in tidy suburban gardens. Yet these may be the very plants on which you will most come to rely for your health and well-being. There is an old saying: A weed is only a plant for which no use has yet been found. Make space for your herbal allies, become friends with plants that turn up uninvited, tune into their virtues, and they will tune in to your needs. We can begin a relationship with plants that will turn in to an extraordinary adventure, inviting engagement with ourselves, our bodies, and our problems at a deep level. *Healing* means "to become whole." We are all called to joy and adventure and to fulfill with cheerfulness and optimism our allotted tasks in life. Plants are our helpers in this endeavor.

Healing is so often about relationships: people become ill or suffer injury when someone dies or when an important relationship is otherwise lost. Anger, jealousy, grief, shock, and disappointment impact energetically on our complex system, and emotions impact directly on our immune competence. Yet how strange and fascinating—and still so little recognized—it is that plants seem to understand our emotions so directly. Honeysuckle gives us courage to plunge into life. The wild rose seems to understand the apathy and despair that settles on those who find life a struggle. In the face of great difficulties, we may give up on life, avoiding challenges and refusing change, surrendering wholly to inertia. The positive and uplifting energies of the wild rose awaken the will, expand the heart and mind, and put us back to work with a sense of purpose and joy.

Such empathy of the plant world with human life is the basis of the Flower Remedies identified by the English physician Dr. Edward Bach (1886–1936). First, he identified the Twelve Healers, and then he defined their Helpers. Flower Remedies are now a worldwide phenomenon, with Australian Bush Essences; Californian, Himalayan, and Alaskan Flower Essences; and many more.

Spagyric Alchemy

Spagyric medicines are prepared in a unique way that captures the full therapeutic spectrum of plants, including the cosmic energies they have absorbed. The method of spagyric preparation has an additional benefit that makes these medicines safer than herbal remedies: in the process of distillation, calcination, and filtration, the heavy metals and other toxins are removed. These are called the *caput mortuum,* or death's head, and are thrown away leaving a purified tincture, or spagyric essence, that is safe to take.

Phytotherapy is based on the idea that there is an energetic or dynamic force in plants that can initiate the recovery of the disturbed life organism in a human being suffering from sickness. Spagyrics, a branch of medicinal alchemy, is one of the oldest methods of extracting and enhancing the energy of plants. It was used and described by Paracelsus, but possibly has much older roots in the applied Hermetic medicinal arts of ancient Egypt.

Roots of Alchemical Philosophy

To appreciate the range and depth of alchemy, we must develop a sympathetic awareness of the spiritual and experiential dimensions of the subject and enter with imagination and sympathy into the worldviews of the past. These are rich, offering glimpses of Egyptian and Hellenistic origins embroidered with Hermetic philosophy and, later fused with Jewish and Christian mysticism. Cosmological and archetypal thinking are an integral part of alchemy. These ideas are often alien to contemporary thought, so dominated by materialism, and yet alchemy is not simply one of the glittering baubles in a basket of rejected knowledge. Alchemy has been the preoccupation of some of the world's greatest minds, from the great Persian physician Avicenna and the giants of twelfth-century science, Albertus Magnus, Roger Bacon, and Robert Grosseteste to Sir Isaac Newton and Robert Boyle in the seventeenth-century scientific revolution. During the early modern period, it was a passionate interest of emperors and princes, physicians, astrologers, musicians, and philosophers. Even the wayward Paracelsus was at one time professor of medicine and city physician in Basel, Switzerland. It is only relatively recently that alchemy has been relegated to the side aisles of history.

Alchemy has its roots in some of the oldest activities of humankind. Among aboriginal peoples, for whom the cosmos is sacred and human work is possessed of liturgical value, working with metals is still regarded as a sacred task. Alchemy has been written about from the second century BCE to the present in all countries of Europe; the Near East; and Persia, India, China, and Tibet. It is clear that alchemy has been, both scientifically and spiritually, a serious pursuit from antiquity to the present. Its roots are in Egyptian metallurgy and priest-craft and in Aristotelian notions of the nature of matter. Without being a religion itself, it has nevertheless been compatible with Jewish mysticism and Kabbalah, and the Christian religion, as well as Neoplatonic, Gnostic, and Hermetic philosophies. It has held fascination for some of the most brilliant and devout minds of every generation. The study of alchemy is now emerging as one of the most exciting interdisciplinary subjects to which linguists, theologians, scientists, and historians of art, literature, music, medicine, psychology, and philosophy can contribute.

Hermes

The mysterious figure of Hermes Trismegistus, a composite of the Egyptian and Hellenistic gods, is the presiding presence in alchemy. The Egyptian god Thoth was associated with the moon, which rules the tides and seasons. His attribute is the ibis, a white bird associated with the moon and with the Nile. Thoth was also the lawgiver, divine scribe, and inventor of writing. The center of the cult of Thoth was at Hermopolis Magna (al-Ashmunayn), once venerated as the oldest place on earth, so Thoth was believed to have played a part in the drama of creation—he was a type of Logos whose voice could call things into being.

Greek settlers in Egypt identified Thoth with their god Hermes, who was son of Zeus and Maia, daughter of Atlas. Hermes' cult was in Arcadia, where he was worshipped as a god of fertility and protector of cattle and sheep. In Homer's *Odyssey,* he appears as the messenger of the gods and psychopomp who conducts the souls of the dead to Hades. In the *Aeneid* (IV, 242), he also goes on a quest to the land of the dead to find people and bring them back to the world of the living. For the living, he was also a dream god, and the Greeks invoked him before sleep. Good luck and casually found treasure were attributed to him. He was celebrated for music, eloquence, prophecy, and divination. In the New Testament, the inhabitants of Lystra take St. Paul for Hermes on account of his eloquence. Greeks living in Alexandria began to conflate their god Hermes with the Egyptian Thoth, and he became subsequently Hermes Trismegistus—"thrice great"—and a whole literary constellation grew around this key figure, chief of which is the *Emerald Tablet* and the *Corpus Hermeticum.*

The Arabs also had a Hermes figure in Idris, the Qur'anic prophet. Idris was a civilizing hero and initiator into the mysteries of the divine sciences and the wisdom that animates the world. He is thought to have carved the sacred science into stone in the form of hieroglyphs. A second Hirmis lived in Babylon and was the legendary initiator of Pythagoras. A sixth-century Arabic text, *The Book of Crates,* mentions a Hirmis who lived before the Flood. According to the text, he foresaw the coming disaster and built the pyramids in which to enshrine the secret knowledge of the world. The *Picatrix,* an Arabic text dating from perhaps the tenth century, describes him as the founder of a city that has not yet yielded up all its marvelous secrets. Such stories demonstrate the creative mix that inspired the Arab imagination, combining Egyptian lore and historical settings with Greek philosophy and myth.[1]

Alexandrian Hermeticism and Alchemy

Through the long Middle Ages, the name Hermes, whether or not qualified as Trismegistus, came to signify a kind of guarantee of authentic knowledge for a host of books on magic, astrology, medicine, and, of course, alchemy, among other esoteric subjects. The so-called Hermetic tradition draws together many ideas from Pythagoreanism, Platonism, Neoplatonism, and some aspects of Gnosticism, and led to a kind of mysticism that expressed itself through natural symbols and the notion of sympathetic correspondence among particular planets, plants, and metals. Over the centuries, this idea of the sacredness of nature promoted Hermeticism to a central role as a cosmological complement to the Christian revelation.

Alexandria, the greatest cultural center of the Hellenistic world, combined Greek, Middle Eastern, and Egyptian influences in an extraordinary, dynamic syncretism, thereby fertilizing many aspects of knowledge and cultural life. During the first three centuries CE, mythic and Neoplatonic ideas blended together to form the beginnings of a philosophy of nature of which the *Corpus Hermeticum* is an example. From this period, Pseudo-Democritus (Bolos of Mendes, the first or second century CE) was already working on a syncretic alchemy. He combined recipes for tinctures with metaphorical and mystical components, ingredients that have colored the understanding of alchemy through the centuries and which were more fully elaborated upon as alchemical allegory by Zosimos of Panopolis (about 300 CE).

In Zosimos's writings we see the development of a *universe imaginaire,* or soul world, that has its genesis in metalworking but goes beyond it into a changed world of meaning. In contrast with earlier texts, which emphasize technical processes, Zosimos presents alchemy as an allegory of the spiritualization of the human being. From this point onward, even though alchemy undoubtedly contributed to technical innovation, it had already ceased to be merely a kind of protochemistry. It opened a door into an altogether more mystical world in which alchemists embarked upon a more ambitious task: the transformation of their own spiritual being and, with it, nature. The acceptance of the essential unity of the universe and the cousinhood of all things in nature opened up an experience of the world that was very different from technical prescriptions. Alchemical work became an immersion in a sacramental activity, and it was termed the Great Work in which prayer and contemplation played an essential part.

Alchemy has three components, which are more or less emphasized at different times: (1) gold as a symbol of highest purity in matter and, usually, the proposition that gold can be produced from baser metals; (2) a search for a universal panacea or elixir that is capable of prolonging life or even conferring immortality; (3) a mystical or redemptive soteriology.

Gold is a kind of absolute symbol expressive of an inward reality ("she has a heart of gold") as well as an outward quality or highest principle, such as the sun or the king who is crowned with gold. In ancient Babylonia, gold was associated with the sun and the god Enlil, and silver was associated with the moon and the god Anu. These associations of gold with the sun and silver with the moon have remained a constant in alchemical iconography throughout its entire history.

Ores and metals were considered to be living things that grew in the womb of the earth. According to alchemical thought, they have gestation and growth within the earth and are ripening toward their perfection as gold. In transmuting baser metal, the alchemists saw themselves as hastening this natural process and performing the godlike task of bringing it to perfection. That which would take thousands of years within the telluric matrix could be brought into being in days or weeks by means of the alchemist's fire. This was not seen as working against nature, for it is nature's purpose to work toward perfection in all things.

In combination, gold and silver, or Sulphur and Mercury, are spoken of as conjoined in a marriage. Though this marriage mirrors that of the union of male and female, usually portrayed as king and queen, it is also conveys a cosmological dimension. It is the mystical union between two cosmological principles and their earthly parallels in metals.

Corpus Hermeticum

This is the primary source for Hermetic philosophy, or Hermetism. The texts are preserved in Greek and are thought to have come originally from Alexandria. When a Byzantine monk, Leonardo of Pistoia, brought a manuscript to Cosimo de' Medici, ruler of Florence, in 1460, it was considered a work more venerable than that of Moses or Plato. Later scholarship has dated the written versions to somewhere between the first and third centuries CE, but its content may be much older and may have existed for centuries in oral form before being written. Some concepts, such as the emanation of man from God likened to the emanation of rays of sunshine from the sun, seem to derive from ancient Egypt. The notion of an archetypal man may derive from esoteric Judaism. As we might expect of a work coming out of Alexandria at the beginning of the Christian era, the *Corpus Hermeticum* combines Hellenistic and Gnostic ideas with Egyptian cosmology and myth and Judaic esoteric mysticism.

We can understand Cosimo de' Medici's impatience to have

Marsilio Ficino translate the work—even before he completed his work on Plato—for the *Corpus Hermeticum* has the tone of a divine revelation, comparable to the book of Genesis. It stresses the living nature of the cosmos (especially Books IX and XIII) and proposes that there is nothing in the cosmos that is not alive. However, the cosmos is not the source of life, but rather God, the Good, or the One.

The other major and radical teaching in the *Corpus Hermeticum* is that the individual human being is also divine—but only if he or she follows the path of spiritual ascent. It is emphasized that this path of *gnosis* cannot be achieved by the ordinary, everyday rational mind. It demands nothing less than a transformation in consciousness: opening to the mystery of revelation using the active organs of true vision, the heart, and the imagination, with which we can slot ourselves back into the ceaseless unfolding of the world that is permanently being created through the divine imagination. Through such a transformation, we can discover the reciprocity of the created world and the human being. All is one. Created and Creator are united in this theophany.

The Hermetic Worldview, or Hermetism

Hermetism is the term given to the doctrine or philosophical perspective described in the *Corpus Hermeticum* in which the scenario of a descent into matter is followed by reintegration and restoration. Hermetism has certain key features that we can recognize as underlying a number of assumptions in alchemy.

Purification of matter and the individual soul is the ultimate goal of the path of Hermetic ascent as one progresses from his or her lower nature to a higher one. The philosophical basis of Hermetism is the mix of Greek nature philosophy and mythology blended with Gnostic and Neoplatonic ideas. Bolos of Mendes, also known as Pseudo-Democritus, provides recipes for tinctures alongside mystical and metaphorical ideas. In his writing about alchemy, Zosimos of Panopolis uses alchemical allegory that has persisted throughout the centuries and has lent itself to the language and interpretation of Christian redemption.

Generally speaking, the first stage in the alchemical process is the regression of matter to its primordial state of chaos: *prima materia.* The substance has to "die" to itself before it can be raised up—which, in alchemy, is brought about either by fire, as in *calcination,* or by being returned to a watery state, as in *dissolution.* This initiatory stage, the preliminary death, is symbolized by darkness or blackness, the *nigredo,* the state of *putrefaction* or *dissolutio.* In alchemy, the quest to raise oneself through purification is mirrored in the operation on matter. St Paul's Epistle to the Romans (8:19–22) describes the Hermetic notion of the human obligation to raise nature as part of our own redemption. Paul asserts that the redemption of nature by human beings is the consummation of the project of redemption of the human world that was initiated by Christ.

Key Themes in the *Corpus Hermeticum*

The universe is a "book" to be "read": we know the Creator God through contemplation of his creation. The universe is full of the manifestation of God, and with our divine intellect, we can decipher the symbols that point toward God. Therefore, we should be interested in everything that is in the world, for the concrete and the particular cannot be displaced. Incarnation and embodiment are ways of experiencing and acting in the world. Our incarnation and embodiment enables us to work in the world on behalf of the unmanifest Creator. As the *Corpus Hermeticum* says: "This is God, greater than a name. He is unmanifest, yet He is most manifest. He can be perceived by *Nous.* He can be seen by the eyes. He is bodiless, yet He has many bodies, or rather every body."[2]

There is an absence of dualism here on earth. The world is recognized as being of divine origin. There is acceptance of the world. Even though we may be pessimistic or discouraged about the consequences of the Fall on the state of humans and nature, this is not the final situation. There is hope of amelioration and restoration through the Hermetic project.

The Hermetic project is one of transmutation of all that is lower, baser, and more material into what is higher, finer, and more spiritual. We are called to this work of regeneration, reascension, and reintegration not only for ourselves, but also to redeem nature. Because we are connected to both divine and earthly worlds, we are able to assist the earth to return to its former glorious state and are ourselves able to return to divinity: "*Nous* is not separate from God's true essence, but is, as it were, spread out from it just like the light of the sun. In men this *Nous* is God, thus some men are gods, and then humanity is akin to divinity."[3]

Our intellects can connect to intermediary spiritual intelligences and use them as rungs in a spiritual ladder. The *Corpus Hermeticum* suggests a belief in an astrological cosmos that, rather than being confined to a form of divination, is part of the initiatory process. The earth is part of this cosmos, and humankind is the microcosm: "God is the soul of eternity; eternity of the cosmos; and heaven of earth. God is in *Nous, Nous* in the soul, soul in matter; and all these things exist through eternity. From within the soul fills this whole body, which contains all bodies, itself being filled by *Nous* and by God."[4]

The mind becomes what it contemplates, hence the importance of the symbolic image and the role of the *mundus imaginalis* as a facilitator of the soul's progress.

Emerald Tablet

Besides the *Corpus Hermeticum* itself, another text of central importance to the philosophy of alchemy is the *Emerald Tablet*. The oldest known version of this text dates from the eighth century and was discovered by E. J. Holmyard, inserted in the *Second Book of the Element of the Foundation*,[5] a book purportedly by the Arab alchemist Jabir ibn Hayyan. This text contains a description of Balinus (i.e., Apollonius of Tyana) finding an engraved tablet in the tomb of Hermes. This legend claims the tablet was written in Phoenician characters and was held in the hands of Hermes' corpse. Philostratus (ca. 170–245) wrote an account of the life of Apollonius, and in Syria, many tales were circulated about the rivalry between this thaumaturge and Hermes. In the *Book of the Secrets of Creation,* written between the sixth century and the mid-eighth century, the names of Apollonius and Hermes are associated.

Though the *Emerald Tablet* was written in Arabic, it is thought to be a translation of an earlier Greek work. In the twelfth century, it was translated from Arabic into Latin by Hugo of Santalla (*fl.* 1141–45). Many versions and translations followed, but it became widely known only when it was printed in 1541. Sir Isaac Newton (1642–1727) was fascinated by the *Emerald Tablet,* which is sometimes considered to be the heart of alchemy. Over a period of twenty years, he studied it extensively and summed up his findings in a *Commentary* now preserved among his papers at King's College, Cambridge.[6]

Mysterious and enigmatic, these few lines from the *Emerald Tablet* are thought to be the kernel of alchemical philosophy and method: The attempt to make "what is below" like "what is above" represents the Hermetic project.

> *True, without deceit, certain and most true.*
>
> *What is below, is like what is above, and what is above is like that which is below, for the performing of the marvels of the one thing.*
>
> *And as all things were from one thing, by the mediation of one thing: so all things were born of this one thing, by adaptation.*
>
> *Its father is the Sun, its mother is the Moon; the wind carried it in its belly; its nurse is the Earth.*
>
> *This is the father of all the perfection of the whole world.*
>
> *Its power is integral, if it be turned into earth.*
>
> *You shall separate the earth from the fire, the subtle from the gross, smoothly and with great cleverness.*
>
> *It ascends from the earth into the heaven, and again descends into the earth and receives the power of the superiors and inferiors. So thus you will have the glory of the whole world. So shall all obscurity flee from thee.*

This is the strong fortitude of all fortitude: because it will overcome
every subtle thing and penetrates every solid.
Thus was the earth created.
Hence will there be marvellous adaptations, of which this is the
means.
And so I am called Hermes Trismegistus, having three parts of the
Philosophy of the whole world.
What I have said concerning the operation of the Sun is finished.[7]

The Dual Nature of Alchemy

Transmutation is the change of one thing into another thing, and is usually thought of as the change of something lower or baser into another that is higher or purer. *Exoteric alchemy* is concerned with this change in substances, thought of popularly as the transmutation of base metals into precious ones, but its logic can also be applied to the purification of herbs to make medicines. In both cases, the original material has to be purged of all that is heavy and dark, such as the heavy metals and alkaloids that make certain plants poisonous. By analogy, in *esoteric alchemy,* the human soul has to be purified in order to receive the gold of a higher consciousness, and so the two kinds of alchemy are inextricably linked. Transmutation can take place on many levels. It may take place in the mind and heart of the adept, effecting the marriage of two poles of identity, or in the flask, where the marriage of Sulphur and Mercury produces "gold."

Alchemy appears to be both a philosophy and an experimental science; both a practice and a mystical aspiration for an elevation of the alchemist's being, a transmutation of the soul. The inner and outer work mirror each other, with the mystical being applied to the manipulation of matter by means of analogy. With the rise of modern chemistry, the metaphysical meaning of alchemy has been lost. Though alchemical texts may contain valuable insights into chemical processes, to focus only upon those is to lose sight of the meaning and function of alchemy as an induction into the *universe imaginaire* of the spirit.[8] This is not to deny that alchemists were concerned with operations of a physical nature and that artists, cathedral

builders, jewelers, physicians, and chemists owe much to the high technological achievements that resulted from the alchemists' labors. When we
look at alchemical images and symbols or read poems and other texts associated with alchemy, we must keep in mind the two aspects of alchemy. A
mystical text may contain important clues to chemical procedures as well.
It is often claimed that alchemists deliberately hid their knowledge behind
all kinds of ciphers and rhetorical devices in order to maintain secrecy, but
it is also true that the esoteric and exoteric were so deeply entwined in the
minds of the alchemists that possibly these practitioners were not always
conscious of the confusion they were creating.

Alchemists attempted to demonstrate the validity of certain metaphysical propositions by working experimentally on the material plane.
The project was to take a philosophical view of the cosmos and prove it
empirically. The object was perfection, both of matter and of the human
being. The symbol of perfection is gold—metal purged of its impurities
just as the soul is purified by the elimination of evil. In the process of
such purification, the alchemist experiences the transmutation of self
and a new birth or union with the divine. In this respect, alchemy has
some parallels with the notion of sacrament—the outward, visible sign
of an inward, spiritual grace.

Roger Bacon (ca. 1214–1292) describes two sorts of alchemy, speculative and practical (*alkimia operativa*), distinguishing between the making of metals and the more philosophical or speculative art.[9] Alchemists
emphasized one aspect over another according to their own viewpoint.
Often, an alchemical treatise was divided up into theory and practice
(*practica* or *operatio*), with the latter giving detailed recipes. Examples
are Arnau de Vilanova's *Rosarium* and Ramon Llull's *Testament*. On
the other hand, Rhazes's *Practica*, Michael Scot's *Alchemia*, the *Alkimia
minor* of Albertus Magnus, and *Liber lucis* of John of Rupescissa (Jean
de Roquetaillade) are concerned more with practical work than theory.
Yet many alchemical works cannot be categorized so easily because
detailed imagery and symbolic language were used to conceal real recipes and methods from the uninitiated.

Alchemy and the Planets

One of the most mysterious aspects of alchemy is the identification of the planets with metals, days of the week, herb plants, and parts of the body. The association of the planets with the metals mercury, gold, silver, iron, copper, lead, and tin seems to go back at least to early Babylonian times and so actually predates any sources we have for alchemy. The correlation of these metals to planets seems to have been present in alchemy from its beginnings. In the Leyden Papyrus (late third century), the sun and moon are used to denote gold and silver. In his *Contra Celsum* (ca. 248), Origen (ca. 185–254 CE) reports on a work by Celsus that describes the "ladder of Mithra." The rungs of this ladder are composed of the planetary metals, and each rung is associated with one of the planetary gods (though the associations are not exactly those that have become traditional).[10]

In the *Timaeus,* Plato describes the stars and planets as visible images of the deities. This is one reason for studying the heavens. For Plato, though, there was also in the heavens a supreme mathematical perfection, a harmony of symmetry, which he took as proof of the manifestation of divine reason. Therefore, he urged any philosopher to study astronomy as the acme of timeless order, perfection, and wisdom. On earth, it seems that everything is subject to change, growth, and decay—a continual process of death and renewal. By contrast, according to Plato, the fixed stars presented a model of eternal stability and regularity, an ordered state that was luminous, timeless, transcendent—a fit dwelling place for the gods.

For the purposes of alchemy, the planetary system remains the Aristotelian-Ptolemaic one that dates from the second century. According to this notion, the earth is the center of the universe from which rise the Four Elements: earth, water, air, and fire. Earth constitutes the sublunary realm or realm of changeability. Above this is the superlunary, celestial, and unchanging world. Here exist the planets in order: Moon, Mercury, Venus, Sun, Mars, Jupiter, Saturn. Above the planets are the fixed stars. The *Corpus Hermeticum* (Book I) suggests that in the individual's incarnational journey, the soul travels down through the planets, collecting their qualities on the way. At death, the soul returns via the planets, relinquishing the vices associated with the planets that have been acquired during the sojourn upon the earth. For example, Mars provides the quality of power, a certain degree of assertiveness with which to act in the world. But this Mars energy can easily turn into its negative pole of mindless aggression.

The planets control the days of the week, and each day is further divided into planetary hours. To the practicing alchemist, it was of great importance to begin the work at the optimal moment, at a time when celestial opportunity would favor the particular phase of the work. Thus, for example, the ideal time to make a plant tincture from a sun plant such as rosemary would be at the sun hour—mid-morning on Sunday.

PLANETARY CORRESPONDENCES

Planet	Symbol	Metals	Elemental Qualities	Days	Planetary Hours	Parts of Body	Zodiac
Sun	☉	Gold	Hot and dry	Sunday	10:17 a.m. to 1:42 p.m.	Heart	Leo
Moon	☽	Silver	Cold and moist	Monday	Midnight to 3:25 a.m.	Brain	Cancer
Mars	♂	Iron	Hot and dry	Tuesday	1:42 p.m. to 5:08 p.m.	Blood	Aries and Scorpio
Mercury	☿	Mercury (Quicksilver)	Cold and dry (masculine); cold and moist (feminine)	Wednesday	3:25 a.m. to 6:51 a.m.	Lungs	Gemini and Virgo
Jupiter	♃	Tin	Warm and moist	Thursday	5:08 p.m. to 8:30 p.m.	Liver	Sagittarius and Pisces
Venus	♀	Copper	Warm and moist	Friday	6:51 a.m. to 10:17 a.m.	Kidney	Taurus and Libra
Saturn	♄	Lead	Cold and dry	Saturday	8:30 p.m. to 12 midnight	Spleen	Capricorn and Aquarius

Planetary Influence on Terrestrial Things

At the beginning of the twentieth century, Lily Kolisko (1889–1976) investigated the behavior of planetary metals during a cosmological event such as a conjunction or opposition of the relevant planets. Using metal salts in solution and a research method known as *capillary dynamolysis,* she was able to determine that a distinct chemical change ocurred in the metals during the Sun-Saturn conjunction of 1926.[11]

Working with capillary dynamolysis is an easy method and shows remarkable results. It can be used for astrochemistry—that is, to show that planets do affect metals on earth—but it is also a way of producing pictures that give a sense of the energetic quality of spagyric tinctures. The experiments call for solutions of mineral salts: sulfate of iron (*Ferrum sulphuricum*), nitrate of silver (*Argentum nitricum*), and lead nitrate (*Plumbum nitricum*). To obtain a solution, 1 gram of pure metallic salt is dissolved in 100 cubic centimeters of distilled water.

The green *Ferrum sulphuricum* salts dissolve rapidly, and the water becomes pale yellow and cloudy. A small amount of light yellow sediment may be deposited in the bottom of the flask. The salts of *Argentum nitricum* dissolve extremely rapidly, and the water appears unchanged in color. *Plumbum nitricum* dissolves very slowly, and again the liquid remains clear. Filter papers dipped into these solutions and allowed to dry show very little at first: the iron sulfate produces merely a fine, wavy brown horizontal line, and the lead nitrate produces almost nothing. The silver nitrate, however, produces a dark, wavy line with some lines descending from it.

Next, equal parts of silver nitrate and iron sulfate solution are added to the filter paper, which has absorbed the lead nitrate. After about a quarter hour, strange forms emerge on the filter paper. Lily Kolisko did these experiments repeatedly, at all times of the day and night, and found that the "rising pictures" (in German, *Steigbilder*) showed distinctive patterns. The forms were strongest at night and quite different from the experiments performed in a darkened room during the day.

Lily Kolisko's major experiment, which appears to show the planetary forces at work on metals, was made on November 21, 1926. At noon on that day, there was an upper conjunction of the Sun and Venus. Later in the day, at 6 p.m. (1800 hours), there was a conjunction of the Sun and Saturn. At this time, Kolisko prepared filter papers from solutions of silver nitrate and lead nitrate.

The results were negligible: none of the characteristic forms manifested on the filter papers. Kolisko continued the experiments throughout the night. She comments:

> Every possible defect in the carrying out of the experiment was guarded against. . . . Yet what did we see? Instead of heavy, massive forms, an utter blank. An invisible hand had blotted out the working of the lead in my solution. And whose was the invisible hand? It was the Sun—the Sun had stood before the planet Saturn and here below on earth the lead could not manifest its activity.[12]

By 11 a.m. on November 22, 1926, the conjunction was over; normal conditions had returned, and the rising pictures again produced the clear characteristic forms. Using Lily Kolisko's method, Theodore Schwenk was able to repeat the experiment over the Mars-Saturn conjunction of 1949. Further experiments by Agnes Fyfe and Nick Kollerstrom have also yielded some persuasive results.[13]

Doctrine of Signatures

In the *Corpus Hermeticum, Nous* teaches Hermes that the mind becomes what it contemplates and that knowledge of God can be obtained by contemplation of the world. God himself is unknowable directly, because he is unmanifest, but nevertheless he can be perceived through his creation, by which he is made manifest. The adept reflects upon the universe in his own spirit and attempts to imprint it within his own psyche. We humans are capable of this because our intellect is a reflection of God; we possess a small bit of *Nous,* which is a reflection of God's greater *Nous.* Characterizing the universe is a web of analogical and dynamic relationships between the lesser and the greater worlds, the macrocosm and the microcosm. Mirror symbolism is widely used in alchemical literature to reaffirm this point.

The most important relationships for the purposes of alchemy are those among the seven planets and the seven metals, and among the planets, the metals, and the organs of the human body. Herbs too may have affinities with one or more of the planets and organs of the body, and this determines their medicinal use. This theory of correspondences was the stimulus for much experimentation. Related to this was the notion of divine seals in nature, or the *doctrine of signatures:* a belief that God has distributed the virtues in plants so that that they can be found by their characteristics. Thus a plant that looks like an eye, such as *Euphrasia,* commonly called eyebright, for example, will be good medicine for eye troubles. A plant that produces a red oil or a red tincture, such as *Hypericum,* was thought to be good for the blood. To see these things in the created world requires that we look not only with the eyes but also with the inner eye, to see things as God sees them.

Salt, Sulphur, and Mercury: Body, Soul, and Spirit

As stated earier, the long therapeutic history of spagyrics can be traced back to the work of the great Swiss-Swabian physician, magus, and alchemist Paracelsus. The term *spagyrics* refers specifically to a branch of plant alchemy in which therapeutic herbs are separated by distillation into their constituent virtues: essential oil, alcohol, and water-soluble salts (electrolytes). Paracelsus regarded these three virtues as the three philosophical principles or *tria prima* of Sulphur, Mercury, and Salt. Obviously, these terms do not refer to the modern elements of the Periodic Table. Instead, they relate respectively to the essential oils, naturally occurring plant alcohols, and water-soluble salts of the plant. These are the soul, spirit, and body of the plant. In therapeutic use, these correspond to the soul, spirit, and body of the individual.

Spagyrics is essentially holistic therapy that works on these three levels of a human being. Once the essential oils, naturally occurring alcohols, and water-soluble salts have been separated and purified, they are then recombined and circulated. This raises the vibration of the spagyric *magistery*. This enhanced energetic quality means that spagyric essences are very fine, perhaps closer to homeopathy than to herbalism. They can be distinguished from herbal remedies because they are more energetic and include the soul and spirit qualities of the essential oils and alcohols as well as the electrolytes of the water-soluble salts contained in the body of the plant.

The separation, refinement, and recombination of the *tria prima* in an alchemical process formed an integral part of Paracelsus's medical and pharmaceutical thought. Rooted in the Hermetic sciences of the Renaissance was the idea that medicines combining the appropriate balance of these principles could be brought into a dynamic interaction—with the patient as microcosm, linking sulphur, mercury, and salt to the soul, spirit, and body of the human being.

In spagyrics, distillation of the plant releases the essential oils and the alcohol that arise from fermentation. Calcination of the remaining plant followed by filtration to exclude the insoluble salts leaves specific minerals and electrolytes in water-soluble salts. After separating the plant into the *tria prima*—its three principles (i.e., sulphur, or essential oils; mercury, or plant alcohols; and salt, or water-soluble salts), the three are recombined to produce a spagyric essence. These essences differ from most plant tinctures in that the thick residue produced after filtration—and containing heavy metals and toxic matter, called the *caput mortuum*—is discarded, thus ensuring that the spagyric essences are nontoxic. The spagyric motto is *Solve et coagula, et habebis magisterium*—"dissolve and coagulate and you will have the magistery."

Sulphur

Sulphur, being solar and associated with gold, plays an important role in alchemical symbolism as the substance that fixes the volatile or liquid mercury. In alchemical iconography, sulphur is fiery and active and often represented by the red King, which joins in mystic marriage (fixes) with the white Queen (mercury).

In plant alchemy, sulphur is the essential oil, or soul, of the plant. It can be volatile, but if the liquid that remains (after distilling off the ethyl alcohol and volatile essential oils) is evaporated, a thick, viscous, honeylike substance remains. This is the fixed sulphur, which can be calcined further to obtain the "salts of the sulphur."

Mercury

Mercury is feminine and under the influence of the moon. In the adaptation of alchemy to Christian Trinitarian thinking, sulphur and salt are sometimes depicted as the parents of the child mercury, who is the son of the sun and moon. In the *Book of Lambsprinck* (*De lapide philosophico*, 1625), mercury is shown as the Holy Spirit sitting between the Father/sulphur and Christ/salt.

Mercury is always hard to define, as befits its association with an elusive and volatile metal. Sometimes mercury is shown as Hermes, the winged messenger of the gods with the wand of the caduceus, and as such, it represents higher consciousness or spirit. In alchemical iconography, it is often depicted as the dual hermaphrodite because of its ambivalence—it is neither solid nor liquid.

In plant alchemy, mercury is the plant alcohol—ethyl alcohol—that is extracted by fermentation and distillation. Unlike sulphur and salt, ethyl alcohol is anonymous in that it does not carry the character or personality of the plant to the same degree as oils and salts. For most practical purposes, therefore, it is admissible to use a high-strength brandy or cognac, as described in the process on page 99.

Salt

To Paracelsus, salt represented the body, or incarnation. According to his follower Gerard Dorn (ca. 1530–1584), salt was like the inner sun in humans, which shines with the light of nature. For Heinrich Khunrath

(1560–1605), salt was the physical center. In iconography, it is sometimes shown as salt water or the Red Sea, which Carl Jung relates to the baptismal water and the emergence of the fully realized individual being.

In plant alchemy, salt is solid and incombustible. It is made by calcination—the incineration of the plant to white ash, which is then added to distilled water. This liquid is then filtered, evaporated, and crystallized several times until a pure white salt is produced. Each plant produces its own individual and unique crystal structure, its own signature, rather like the unique patterns made by snowflakes.

The Magistery

Spagyric preparations include the whole plant, and, because of the special processes that both purify and slightly energize or potentize them, they offer enhanced healing power that is truly holistic. Separation reveals the philosophical trinity posited by Paracelsus: the body, soul, and spirit of the plant is present in them. By recombining them, a spagyric remedy becomes greater than the sum of its parts and is easily assimilated. It can be used to stimulate autoregulation (homeostasis) and for prophylaxis.

Spagyric essences differ from Flower Remedies and aromatherapy oils (which contain only sulphur) because they incorporate the salt (body of the plant), from which toxic matter has been purged. Spagyric essences also differ from normal herbal tinctures because such tinctures may still retain the toxic, insoluble salts, which spagyric calcination and filtration exclude. Individual spagyric essences are selected according to homeopathic principles, but they can also be combined on the basis of general phytotherapeutic (herbalist) practice. Spagyrics differ from homeopathic remedies because, although they are energized (very slightly potentized) by circulation, they are not diluted at successive stages as homeopathic remedies are. Yet there have been some experiments to make homeopathic remedies from spagyric essences, and some spagyric pharmacies do this, claiming that Kirlian photography, electroacupuncture screening, point-testing, and other types of analysis all show a higher inherent energy quotient in homeopathic-spagyrics.[14]

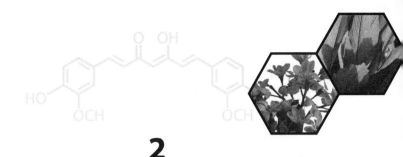

2

Paracelsus

The pioneer of medicinal alchemy was the colorful sixteenth-century physician Paracelsus (1493–1541), a major figure in the history of Western esotericism. His work was a turning point in alchemical theory and practice. He pioneered important changes in medical practice, and he was an original theological thinker whose ideas were the basis of a posthumous Theophrastia Sancta or Paracelsian religion among the many post-Reformation marginal spiritual groups.[1] He was also an inspiration for the Rosicrucian movement. Above all, this charismatic figure had a lasting influence on alchemy and medicine, inaugurating both homeopathy and chemical medicine (*iatrochemistry*). His ideas of medicine are inextricably linked to his understanding of the subtle aspects of the human body and the nature of healing.

Despite the extent of his influence, little is really known for certain about Paracelsus. Andrew Cunningham has drawn attention to the "thin Paracelsus"—that is, what is known from his own lifetime—and the "fat Paracelsus," which is what has been made of him posthumously.[2] In recent years, he has been the object of impressive scholarly studies.[3] There are also numerous popular accounts of his life, more or less embroidered depending on the temperament and imagination of the biographer.[4]

Philippus Aureolus Theophrastus Bombastus von Hohenheim* was born in Einsiedeln on November 11, 1493. Then as now, Einsiedeln was a place of piety and pilgrimage. St. Meinrad, a Benedictine monk from Reichenau on Lake Constance, set up a hermitage there around 835. St. Meinrad brought with him a small statue of the Virgin Mary made for Hildegarde of Zurich. It was claimed that this statue had miraculous powers, and it established Einsiedeln as a center of Marian pilgrimage. It remains so to this day, and is one of the four hundred or so sites in Europe dedicated to veneration of the Black Virgin. As in everything else, Paracelsus had his own idiosyncratic view of the sacraments and doctrines of the church. The piety in Einsiedeln surrounding the Virgin Mary, which he would have known since his childhood, may be the root of the elevated status of Mary as the celestial queen and bride of God in Paracelsus's religious thought.[5]

Paracelsus was born into a world already in a dramatic surge of change. The tone was set by the discovery of the New World in 1492 and was carried forward in the search for new horizons in every aspect of life, belief, and scholarship. Charles Webster has noted the importance of contextualizing Paracelsus's life within the turmoil of the Reformation, even though Paracelsus himself did not align himself with any schismatic group, instead desiring a unified and spiritually based church.[6] During his lifetime, Paracelsus was called the Luther of Medicine, and his birth was framed by those reformers in the last decades of the fifteenth century and the first decade of the sixteenth—from Oecolampadius and Luther, born in 1482 and 1483, respectively, to Calvin in 1509.

The older Desiderius Erasmus (ca. 1466–1536), with whom Oecolampadius worked on the Greek New Testament, fired an opening salvo of the Reformation with his book *In Praise of Folly* (1509), which lampoons the clergy and the more superstitious aspects of the Roman

---

*The name Paracelsus was a nickname taken later by Philippus Aureolus Theophrastus Bombastus von Hohenheim, see page 37.

Catholic faith. Huldreich Zwingli (1484–1531) was one of the first of the younger generation to lead reform from Einsiedeln, publishing against the corruption of the church in 1516, a year before Luther posted his ninety-five theses on the door of Wittenberg Church. Zwingli had gone to Einsiedeln to meditate and consider his position with regard to reform, and it was in Paracelsus's hometown that he made his decisive choice, reacting powerfully against the corruption in the church and the veneration of the Virgin Mary as well as against other aspects of the church that he regarded as superstitious beliefs. The questioning of old authorities and orthodoxies was very much in line with Paracelsus's own mind-set; he was most at home with dissenters, free-thinkers, and rebels, though he never wavered from his belief in the Christian faith, nor did he break away from the Roman Catholic church.

Paracelsus was born midway between the births of two other leading pioneers of the age who also changed the world of their time in ways that were to have far-reaching effects: twenty years after Copernicus (1473–1543) and before Van Wesele "Vesalius" (1514–1564). Their two ground-breaking publications—Copernicus's *De revolutionibus orbium coelestium* (1543) and Vesalius's *De humani corporis fabrica* (1543)—saw the light of day just two years after Paracelsus's death in Salzburg on September 24, 1541. Allen G. Debus comments that "the significance of his [Paracelsus's] opening of medical thought to this new approach [academic acceptance of chemistry by physicians] can be compared with that of Copernicus on astronomy and physics during the same period."[7] In the long run, Vesalius's *De fabrica* assisted in the shift away from passive reliance upon Galen as the major medical authority, something Paracelsus had been eager to achieve.

The intellectual world in which Paracelsus lived comprised the divided worlds of the Reformation and Renaissance humanism, and was characterized by a search in newly recovered classical texts for clues to life and knowledge in all of its aspects. Ancient authors were examined in a new light in the search for new patterns to follow in literature and rhetoric. Humanist writers now strove to write in stylish and polished

Latin that would outshine the "barbarous" Latin of the Middle Ages. By the late fifteenth century, the recovery of ancient of texts had also begun to affect science. Ptolemy's *Almagest,* which many thinkers relied upon for both mathematics and astronomical observations, fostered an increased interest in science and laid the foundations for Copernicus's *De revolutionibus orbium.*

Above all, the humanist project was centered on both the relatively newly acquired knowledge of Greek, which was due, in no small part, to the visit of Gemistos Plethon (ca. 1355–1450) to the court of Cosimo de' Medici in 1439, and the setting up of the Platonic Academy under Marsilio Ficino (1433–1499) at the Villa Carreggi. Rather than relying on much-translated works of the Middle Ages (from Greek into Syriac, from Syriac into Arabic, from Arabic into Latin), with the revival of Greek learning, scientists examined the original Greek sources of medicine— chiefly Hippocrates and Galen—for a pure stream of ancient medicine. In addition to these "fathers of medicine"—Hippocrates and Galen—the work of the encyclopedist Celsus (ca. 25 BCE–50 CE), *De medicina,* the elegant Latin source of Alexandrian medical knowledge, was printed in Florence in 1478. At first, the recovery of these ancient medical sources led to their entrenchment among the medical elite—yet there was consternation about the many areas of disagreement in the text, and attempts were made to build a complete edifice from the scattered works of Aristotle, Galen, the herbalist Dioscorides, Avicenna, and Hippocrates that stressed their commonalities rather than their differences. Symphorien Champier was one of the scholars who sought to merge these works. His *Symphonia Platonis cum Aristotle, et Galeni cum Hyppocrate* (Paris, 1516) sought to reconcile the ideas of the great philosophers and the fathers of medicine.

In the inquiring decades of the early sixteenth century, however, Greek texts were examined more searchingly. When Vesalius, a Greek scholar, professor of anatomy at Padua, came to research anatomy, he went back to Galen in the original Greek just as he also undertook dissection himself, examining the body against the texts of ancient authorities.

Paracelsus reacted against what he saw as the unwarranted authority of the ancient writers; he believed the sources of knowledge were experience and the "light of Nature." He also reacted against the fashion for ancient languages, preferring to teach and write in German.

We know little about Paracelsus's early life. His father, the illegitimate son of a nobleman, was a practicing alchemist and physician who passed on to Paracelsus a passion for this work. According to legend, Paracelsus may have studied alchemy with Johann Trithemius (1462–1516), whose library contained more than two thousand hand-copied manuscripts and printed books. It may have been through Trithemius that Paracelsus discovered the work of Hildegard of Bingen (1098–1179), who had lived her whole life in the rural Rhineland, in proximity to Sponheim, where Trithemius first became abbot. Trithemius certainly knew her work and had personally copied her manuscripts on medicine and natural history. Her vision of the cosmic egg and the emphasis she placed on the idea of the macrocosm-microcosm have distinct parallels in Paracelsus's thought. Paracelsus also followed Hildegard's position with regard to the stars, which he thought influenced but did not have absolute sway over human affairs.[8]

Paracelsus may have attended medical studies in Vienna and may have obtained a medical doctorate from Ferrara, but this is largely doubted. During the early 1520s, Paracelsus was a wanderer, undertaking an enormous peregrination.[9] He also had a preference for knowledge from unorthodox sources, believing experience to be more important than academic learning. He is often quoted as saying, "The universities do not teach all things," and he himself was prepared to learn from midwives and local people as he traveled across Europe. When it came to knowledge of the created world, Paracelsus believed the Light of Nature was the supreme teacher. According to Paracelsus, the Light of Nature was able to communicate with the spirit of the human being and "no physician can establish the basis of diseases or indeed of the human being without sufficient witnesses from the light of nature. That light is the great world [macrocosm]."[10]

His reputation as a healer spread, eventually reaching the ears of the renowned humanist publisher, Froben, in Basel. When his own doctors could do nothing to save his leg from the threat of amputation, Froben sent for Paracelsus, who accomplished a seemingly miraculous cure. While at Froben's house, Paracelsus met the great humanist scholar Erasmus, whom he also treated. In gratitude, Froben and Erasmus managed to secure for Paracelsus the prestigious linked posts of city physician at Basel and professor of medicine at Basel University.[11] At this news the numbers of students enrolled in the medical course shot up from five to more than thirty. It was the high point of Paracelsus's public career, but it also contained the seeds of his downfall.

Paracelsus had always lambasted academics and was completely unsuited to the etiquette of academe. He refused to lecture in Latin, supposing he would make himself better understood in the vernacular. In a lecture concerning the health of the bowels as related to the overall health of the patient, he further scandalized the authorities by bringing a bowl of excrement into the lecture room. There must have been a number of such irritants on both sides, and these came to a head on St. John's Day, 1527, when Paracelsus joined in the students' festivities with zeal and famously threw the revered works of Galen and Avicenna onto a bonfire. After a further fracas over a patient refusing to pay his fee, Paracelsus was dismissed and had to flee. From this time forward, he called himself Paracelsus (rather than his given name of von Hohenheim), and he embarked on further wanderings in German lands. He died in Salzburg in 1541.

The sense of going beyond the status quo became Paracelsus's trademark. His own nickname meant "going beyond Celsus," and the titles of his books, such as *Paragranum* [Beyond the Grain] (1528–30) and *Opus Paramirum* [Beyond Wonder] (1531), also reflected this idea of surpassing what had gone before.

Medicine at the Time of Paracelsus

Hippocrates of Cos

The fathers of medicine still revered in Paracelsus's lifetime were Avicenna, Hippocrates, and Galen. Hippocrates of Cos (ca. 460–370 BCE) was the first to free illness from the stigma of punishment by the gods. Rather than believing illness was divine retribution, he believed it was more likely the result of poor diet and unhealthy living habits. He recommended gentle medicine and a wholesome regime based upon clean water, good food, rest, and recreation. He began to use the pulse for diagnosis, recognized that cancer more often affected people who were in an unhappy frame of mind than those who had a sunny disposition, and laid the foundations for endoscopy and the treatment of hemorrhoids that is still widely in use today. Above all, he took a "vitalist" view of the body, believing the organism had powerful abilities of recuperation and could heal itself when provided with positive conditions. His remedies were based on the homeopathic notion that "like cures like"—that is, herbs or even poisonous plants that would cause symptoms in a healthy person would cure those same symptoms in the sick. Paracelsus, Samuel Hahnemann, the founder of homeopathy, and the later spagyrists all followed Hippocrates' idea of similarity in the cure of disease.

Galen of Pergamon

Galen (ca. 130–201 or 216) from Pergamon, in Asia Minor—now in Turkey—was the outstanding physician of the Roman Empire. A polymath who combined a love of science with philosophy, he traveled extensively and studied medicine in Smyrna, Corinth, and Alexandria in the early 150s before settling down as physician in Pergamon. For four years, from 162 to 166, he was in Rome as surgeon to the gladiators, but he retreated to obscurity in 166. Marcus Aurelius (121–180) recalled him to Rome two years later, calling him first among physicians.

Galen wrote in Greek, which was translated into Latin in the fifth century. Although much of his work was lost in the fire of the library at Alexandria, the dual language of his works ensured that they would survive through the following centuries. Greek medicine was spread by Nestorian Christian missionaries in their own language, Syriac, until it was assimilated into the Arabic world when Galen's works (in Syriac translation) were translated into Arabic under Hunayn ibn Ishaq of Jundishapur. In 856, Hunayn compiled a list of the 129 works of Galen that were known to him, cataloging them in both Syrian and Arabic versions. Until the Renaissance, when the Greek works emerged from Byzantium, Galen's works were known either in Arabic or in the medieval translations of Arabic into Latin. Constantinus Africanus (d. prior 1098/9), a monk at Monte Cassino, was one of the Latin translators, alongside Gerard of Cremona and the Toledo school of translators. By the fourteenth century, these translations had established Galen in every medical school in Europe, and, despite controversy, his dominance persisted, in some places even into the nineteenth century.

Galen's medicine, based on the four humors, derived ultimately from Aristotle's elaboration of the four-element theory of Empedocles. Empedocles, a poet, attributed all cause to the immaterial principles of love and strife, which worked with the four elements of fire, air, earth, and water. These elements, which Empedocles personified as the gods Zeus, Hera, Aidoneus, and Nestis, were the roots from which "sprang all things that were and are and shall be; trees and men and women, beasts and birds and water-bred fishes, and the long-lived gods too, most mighty in their prerogatives. For there are these things alone, and running through one another they assume many a shape."[12] Brought together by love and dispersed again by strife, a continual process of binding and loosening, the elements whirling in a cosmic dance brought all into being and separated them again. Alchemical theory came to rest entirely on the four elements until queried by Paracelsus, van Helmont, and Robert Boyle. Medical theory also depended on the qualities of the four elements—hot, dry, cold, and moist—that Galen related to the four humors of the human constitution. Another insight from Empedocles—"like can only be known by like, only nature can understand itself, only nature can fathom itself, but only spirit can also understand spirit"—also had a long-lived career in Paracelsus's ideas of the microcosm and the notions of Samuel Hahnemann, who took it as a fundamental principle of homeopathy.[13]

In *De elementis de temperamentis* and the fragment *De facultatum naturalium substantia,* Galen set out the relationship among the elements (humors) of the human body—blood, phlegm, and black and yellow bile—and of nature (earth, air, fire, and water). He suggested a *symmetron*—a point of balance in an individual or in a species—between the extremes of temperament. Thus the *eucraton,* or ideal temperament, is one in which the activity of each element is in equal proportion to all the others. This equilibrium can be perceived by the perfection of health and activity in an individual or species. Disease is, therefore, the result of a breakdown in this equilibrium.[14] Galen and his followers believed health derived from a proper balance of the four humors, while disease resulted from imbalance. The humors were perceived by sensory evaluation of the patient, mostly following obvious visual clues, such as an excess of blood as evidenced by a florid complexion or phlegm evidenced by a runny nose. In medical diagnosis, it was thought that the skin of the patient registered the temperament through the sensible qualities, and also that the skin of the fingertips was uniquely favored for the careful discernment of the equilibrium between hot and cold, moist and dry—literally a hands-on approach to diagnosis.[15]

An anatomist at Bologna, Thaddeus of Florence (1223–1303), was one of the first to recognize the importance of starting afresh with Greek texts. The medicine, surgery, and anatomy of Bologna were of Arabic origin, and they in turn were transplanted to Montpellier by a Bologna alumnus, Henri de Mondeville (1270–1320), when he moved to the south of France in 1301.[16] Along with Paris, Bologna and Montpellier became the leading medical faculties, with more minor ones at Padua, Ferrara, and Oxford.

In the fifteenth and sixteenth centuries, in the intense activity surrounding the recovery of ancient medical texts led by Johannes Guinther of Andernach (1487–1574), Galen emerged as the leading medical authority. The certainty of his tone and the dogmatic style of his works were partly responsible for Galen's enduring legacy. By 1500, there were several translations of Galen's *De usu partium,* and the collected works appeared in Greek in 1525. Andernach, who translated Galen's *De anatomicis admistrationibus* (1531), was assisted by his pupil Andreas Vesalius (1514–1564), who would finally demote Galen from his preeminence with *De humani corporis fabrica* (1543). Thomas Linacre (ca. 1460–1524), physician to King Henry VII and King Henry VIII of England and founder of the Royal College of Physicians (1518), who had learned both his medicine and his Greek in Padua, instituted major translation programs of Galen, bringing out *De naturalibus facultatibus* in 1523.[17]

The correction of humors involved great discomfort for the patient; it became known as the "heroic" method, for it involved violent periods of purging, emetics, sweating, and above all, bloodletting, a practice that still survives. Galen had introduced such novelties as diagnosis from dreams, but this was a very simple and literal concept: if an individual dreamed of snow, the medical indication was a shivery condition; if an individual dreamed of a leg turned to stone, the medical indication was real or incipient paralysis.

Paracelsus did not know Greek, but he felt an antipathy toward Galen on several counts. Broadly speaking, he inclined toward the vitalist notions of Hippocrates. He knew from experience the success of the homeopathic principle of "like cures like," declaring that "what makes a man ill also cures him," but he also anticipated the homeopathic dilution: "All things are poison, and nothing is without poison. The amount alone decides that a thing is not poison." Though "contraries" also had an undeniable therapeutic pedigree, Paracelsus joined in the reaction against humoral medicine that had begun with the arrival of the Black Death in 1348–49. Balancing the humors was a long-term project, but the plague killed in a matter of days—thus other approaches had to be tried.[18]

Though in the later Middle Ages and early Renaissance there was no decisive break with the medicine of the early Middle Ages and its steadfast reliance on classical and Islamic sources, nevertheless the period 1200–1600 can be viewed as a distinct era in the history of medicine. It was during these centuries that medicine was instituted as a discipline within the emerging universities, with Montpellier and Bologna (1156) leading the field. With the twelfth-century translations from Arabic into Latin, alchemy began to play a major role in the search for medicines.[19]

The notion of a medicine that would confer long life and rejuvenation surfaced early in the thirteenth century in a treatise *De retardatione accidentium sectutis,* attributed to Roger Bacon, which appeared in the papal court. Underpinning Roger Bacon's innovative ideas relating to alchemy and pharmacology was a doctrine of separation whereby the alchemist might take elementary bodies back to their unitary root, or *prima materia,* and unite them again in a more balanced mix. He is perhaps the first of all English alchemists to describe the spagyric method as a means of perfecting medicines. The separations of medicinal virtues, he says, "can only be properly effected by alchemical methods, which alone teach how active principles are extracted from certain things. For in remedies there should be solutions and separations of one thing from another thing, and this can only be done by the power of alchemy. . . . Examples are infinite, for instance, in the case of phlegm-purging rhubarb the active principle should be taken without the gross substance, a thing of which almost the whole medical world is ignorant."[20] In the fourteenth-century *Rosarium Philosophorum,* attributed to Arnau of Vilanova (1235–1315), such medicine has a "more active virtue than every other remedy, because of its occult and subtle nature."[21]

Paracelsus's Theory of Disease

If the humoral model did not fit with the treatment of plague, Paracelsus argued, it was also useless with regard to the relatively recent emergence of hither-to-unknown diseases such as syphilis. Nor did it fit with the occupational diseases Paracelsus had identified among miners.

Moreover, Paracelsus had a much more complex picture of the causes of disease, which he argued were five in number: *Ens Astrorum* (historical/cosmological); *Ens Naturale* (constitutional); *Ens Veneni* (toxicity); *Ens Spirituale* (imagination, fear, or phobia); and *Ens Dei* (at the will of God, or purgatorial diseases). This last idea had been prevalent in early Greek thought, and Hippocrates had gone some way toward rejecting the notion that disease was the punishment of the gods. Yet in the Christian world, the idea came back with force, particularly because the devastating plagues that swept Europe seemed otherwise so inexplicable. Paracelsus believed that every illness was potentially curable. Of course, he posited, not all would be cured; some diseases, the result of the *Ens Dei,* could be relieved only by God, and the patient had to wait for God's own time.

With a wide range of medicines at his disposal that were derived from all three kingdoms—including many substances normally considered poisonous—Paracelsus believed that it was possible to select a medicine that would restore health without correcting the humors. In fact, though, the medicines were less important than the state of the inner physician, which he termed the *archeus.*

In *Paragranum* or *Against the Grain* (1528–30), Paracelsus laid out the four pillars of medical art:

1. Natural Philosophy
2. Astronomy: relations between human and universe
3. Alchemy: knowledge and preparation of medicines
4. Virtue: personal powers latent in the physician and in the herb or metal and in the patient; the archeus

His assertion of the first three pillars "was in line with an entrenched position established by medieval Arabic and Jewish medical authorities, and reflected in the prevailing bias of the medical education of his day."[22] Natural philosophy, mathematics, and astrology were standard components of medical studies while alchemy had a "niche in the study of pharmacology."[23] The closeness of astrology and medicine was evidenced by the fact that Copernicus, Tycho Brahe (1546–1601), and Kepler (1571–1630) were all medically trained and Copernicus's amanuensis and student, Rheticus (1524–1574), was a successful practicing physician. Jean Fernel (1497–1558) was probably the first to propose dispensing with astrology in his *Universa medicina* (1554), much to the consternation of the medical faculty establishment, who considered seeking assistance from the stars as part of the natural order of medical conduct.[24] Astrology was extremely important for venesection. Just as the moon controls the tides, so it also influences blood flow. Physicians recognized that bloodletting at the full moon could be fatal to the patient. For Paracelsus, however, the stars had a special place in medicine because the human being has a cosmic dimension, and "since so much depends upon the heavens . . . its action must be known to a medicine which is so forcefully dominated by them."[25]

Alchemy until the Time of Paracelsus

Constantinus Africanus, a major source of Greek-Arabic science translated into Latin, was influential at Salerno, one of the oldest proto-university institutions in Europe. As the leading center for the reception of Arabic scientific and medical literature, for more than two centuries it remained one of the most progressive medical schools in Europe. It was from here that many recipes for alcohol emerged in the twelfth century and found their way into recipe books such as *Compendium Salerni*—writings from Salerno. Crucially important for medicinal alchemy was the art of distillation, which had been practiced in the West since the twelfth century,[26] but which was made far more popular by the publication of *Liber de arte distillandi de compositis* (Strasbourg, 1512) by the popular surgeon Hieronymous Brunschwyg (1450–1534). At this time, surgeons were somewhat outside the academic bastions of medicine; they had to be apprenticed and were taught techniques first-hand. For this reason, they were often far more progressive than doctors and thus, like Brunschwyg, more receptive to new ideas.[27]

From the twelfth century, alchemy certainly seems to have had a continuous role in the curriculum. Walter Pagel comments that the medical schools had

> ... an unbroken tradition in chemistry, derived partly from the exigencies of commerce and mining and partly from the aspirations of alchemy, as transmitted by Christian, Gnostic and Neo-Platonic syncretism with Oriental ideas. In this connection, we can recall Arnau of Vilanova (ca. 1235–1312) and Roger Bacon (ca. 1214–1292) as well as the proto-scientific element in "Magia Naturalis."[28]

Already, by the late-thirteenth century, the *Liber claritatis* and works attributed to Michael Scot and to the Latin Geber had demonstrated a relatively modern tone in their descriptions of techniques and processes to do with metals and mineral acids, even those of corrosive sublimates of mercury.[29] The Latin Geber was the first to describe the production of nitric acid. Referring to the mineral acids—such as hydrochloric, nitric, and sulfuric acids—Multhauf writes that "it would be difficult to overestimate the impact of the mineral acids on chemical technology."[30] By the middle of the fourteenth century, treatises emerged exploring improved procedures of distillation and mineral acid dissolution.[31]

Arnau of Vilanova had already proposed that alchemy must play a role in the reform of medicine—for how else could an elixir of life be discovered? The plagues beginning in 1348 further stimulated the search for "the mother and Empress of medicines, [which] others have named ... the inestimable glory; others, indeed, have named it the quintessence, the philosophers' stone, and the elixir of life."[32]

At Montpellier, as at Bologna, students studied the teaching of Rhazes and Avicenna (Ibn Sina) in particular, and "from these two centers . . . the teaching and the Islamic culture spread to every medical school in Europe."[33] The teachings of Rhazes and Avicenna remained in use as textbooks at Montpellier until the middle of the sixteenth century, when it became a center for Paracelsian alchemical medicine.[34] Laboratories, with equipment developed from Arab prototypes, belonged to the pharmaceutical tradition of monastic hospitals and "as an extension of university pharmacies in the late Middle Ages, and at princely courts."[35]

Medical studies in England lagged behind those on mainland Europe, and it was usual for students at Oxford and Cambridge to proceed to continental universities to top up their medical education. In the early (Henrician) Tudor period, "the course of study and the required textbooks were similar all over Europe, where the formal lectures were still a strange mixture of alchemy, medicine, magic and astrology."[36]

Yet a major example of the crossover between monastic and university science in England is the Franciscan Roger Bacon, who was not only the most able scientist and mathematician of thirteenth-century Oxford, but also eminent as a medical and alchemical sage, which earned him the soubriquet *Doctor Mirabilis*.[37] Although it is not clear that Bacon was a practitioner of medicine, "medical doctors, especially in the Oxford circle, looked to Bacon as a great medical and alchemical theorist."[38] Pereira notes that "alchemy and medicine have been closely linked in the western scientific tradition since the time of Roger Bacon, and their link is the main concern of alchemical writings focusing on the theme of the elixir," of which those attributed to Arnau of Vilanova and Raymond Llull are the most notable.[39]

Certainly alchemy, which had been defined as a science in *Speculum naturale* by Vincent of Beauvais (1190–1264), was discussed at university level by 1300, and scholars would have been familiar with the elixir as described at length by Vincent.[40] In the late-sixteenth and seventeenth centuries, Paracelsian views of medical alchemy were first adopted in those medical centers where there existed already a keen interest in alchemy and practical chemistry.[41]

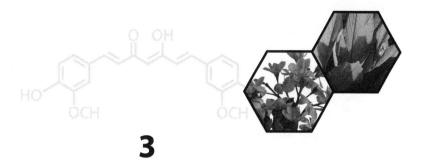

3
Paracelsian Philosophy and Spagyric Alchemy

Medicinal alchemy is not only about laboratory techniques or the knowledge of plants, important though those are. Its animating philosophy, derived from ancient sources but articulated and elaborated more fully in Paracelsus, includes the theory of macrocosm and microcosm; the Hermetic notion of "as above so below"; the astral body; the archeus. On a practical level, we derive from Paracelsus the *tria prima,* or the three principles of Salt, Sulphur, and Mercury. Perhaps the most marked contrast with modern orthodox medicine is that in Paracelsus we find an echo of Plato's dictum that the healing of the body should not be attempted without the healing of the soul. Thus considering the prescription of spagyric medicine entails a holistic view of the patient and attention to the qualities of soul life. Paracelsus repeatedly urges us to meditate upon all these things. He takes it for granted that prescriptions are based upon the homeopathic *similimum,* or like curing like, and that, given the right opportunity, the body heals itself.

Macrocosm and Microcosm in Paracelsus

As Walter Pagel has commented, Paracelsian medicine is based on a "Cosmological Anthropology," which brings together medicine, alchemy, theology, and cosmology.[1] In this respect Paracelsus achieved a successful fusion of Neoplatonic ideas and medicine. Despite his many points of contention with the work of Avicenna (980–1037), Paracelsus nevertheless followed Avicenna's example in making the microcosm the foundation of his theory of medicine. "Since the body is the dwelling place of the soul, the two are connected and the one must open access to the other," he says, directly echoing Plato.[2]

For Paracelsus, the universe was vividly alive with magical forces that are disclosed by the grace of God, through visionary or mystical experience or personal observation, to those who seek knowledge of the universe as a means of finding knowledge of God.

Alchemy was one important clue to understanding the universe by providing an understanding of the elements that make up the cosmos. It was a common alchemical theme that matter had to be regressed to its early stages of creation in order to be transmuted, and this idea was developed in the posthumously published (and possibly pseudepigraphic) *Philosophia ad Athenienses* (1564). Alchemy was also seen as a means to understanding the mind of God, whose own method of creation was deemed to be alchemical. In God's alchemy of creation, which worked with the *mysterium magnum,* separation reduced everything to its own particular essence, and assigned to each essence its own individual form. Spirits were produced by separation from air, water, plants, and salts; creatures that live in water were produced by separation from water; and animals, stones, and plants came from separation from earth. Each created thing was separated from those already created. Thus the elements were the "mothers" of created objects; human beings contain the impression of all created things because they derive from the same mother.[3]

It is therefore incumbent upon the physician to know and understand the world, for only in this way, according to Paracelsus, is he able to come to know and understand his patients:

[People] should know the great human being, pursuing it into the
inner one. . . Unless you ruminate daily on the things I tell you—

how else would you arrive at the foundation of medicine? How else will you get to know the *microcosmos* in external nature, in which you will comprehend wonders and great secret things that reside within the human being.[4]

The pulse can be comprehended from the firmament [or] physiognomy in the stars; . . . the fevers in earthquakes . . . if the physician masters the things externally from word to word, then he sees and knows about all diseases outside the human being. For when the human being with all his conditions has been modeled in this way, [the physician] enters [the realm of] the inner human being: for then you are a physician. Examine, then, the maladies of the human being, feel the pulse, assess the person, and [do so] not without a vast understanding of the external human being, which is nothing other than the heavens and the earth themselves . . .[5]

Paracelsus found parallels between elemental macrocosmic events and the ailments of the human being. Thus thunder was analogous to macrocosmic stroke, precipitation to dropsy; an earthquake to an epileptic fit. The physician can perceive and know these things because the macrocosm is inside his own being.

One who recognized the sun or moon and [who] knows even with closed eyes what they are like, has the sun and moon within him, just as they stand in the heavens and firmament. That is what philosophy is: [things] are in the human being in the same way that they are outside, intangibly, as if one were looking at oneself in a mirror. And [. . .] the physician must bear a precise knowledge of the human being within him, extracted from the mirror of the four elements; [for] the latter present to him the entire *microcosmos* in such a way that [the physician] can . . . look though a human being, just as transparently as if seeing through to a distilled dew in which not even the least little spark could be hidden so that it would remain unseen.[6]

In some respects, Paracelsus's ideas about the parallels between macrocosm and microcosm seem somewhat literal. Yet he also propounded a more magical aspect to the theory whereby the human being can tap into active celestial powers within the macrocosm in order to shape terrestrial events, particularly with regard to human health. Paracelsus developed an alchemical application of the microcosm theory in tandem with his ideas of the method of action of medicines and human relations to the stars. Through the macrocosm, the deep sympathy that obtained among all created things led Paracelsus to suppose that medicinal action was possible at a distance. Paracelsus—and after him, the English physician Robert Fludd (1574–1637)—discussed the weapon salve as capable of producing healing at a distance by treating the knife that had made the wound. This was said to work because of the sympathetic attraction of the stars acting through the intermediary of air. "The cure is done by the magnetique attractive power of this Salve, caused by the Starres, which by the mediation of the ayre, is carried and adjoyned to the Wound, that so the Spirituall operation thereof may bee effected."[7]

Alchemy, a science of relationship, embraces the correspondences between the creation of the cosmos and the Work, and between the Work and the human agent. As Robert Grosseteste (ca. 1170–1253) pointed out, the Aristotelian separation of heaven and earth was repaired in alchemy by the goal of unity.[8] The extraction of noble metals from impure ores requires solvents and purifying agents in conjunction with fire. The unleashing of powerful natural forces paralleled the creation of the world in the beginning, but it extended to the purification of the moral self. Morienus comments that alchemy is an inner process as well as an outer work, and here we find a hint that the first temptation to be resisted is covetousness; the moral threshold begins with materiality. The shaping of human's moral sense begins with his control over matter—but for the alchemist, control over matter begins with the understanding of the cosmic powers latent within him. For Paracelsus, nature and philosophy were inextricably linked: "The physician must be educated by nature. . . . What is nature but philosophy? What is philosophy other than the invisible nature?"[9] Paracelsus, boisterous and assertive as he was, inhabited a world of intangibles in which the operations of occult and magical forces were proximate. As a condensation of the macrocosm, the human being had powers to know and to operate the natural powers at work in creation. This is due to the Hermetic relationship of the above and the below. The stars, he says, are the father of the human being; the elements are the mother. The offspring of a celestial and terrestrial pairing, the human being, possesses a visible mortal body and an invisible immortal one with a special relationship to the stars.

The Astral Body

The *astral body* is an ancient, ambiguous Neoplatonic term mentioned by Porphyry and Proclus. Its general character is thought to be fine, lucent, and subtle and "identical with the substance of the stars and spheres, through which the soul passes while descending from its origin to this earth, or, if not identical, it has received successive celestial influences as imprints during this descent."[10] This idea is similar to that of the Hermetic journey of the soul, which is said to wend through the planets, accruing the planetary virtues on the way, and which returns, after death, through the planets, relinquishing their vices.

Although metempsychosis and preexistence of the soul did not conform to Christian theology, during the early Renaissance there was a powerful and pervasive belief that the heavens contained the forms of all things and distributed them to earth by means of the *spiritus mundi,* and that nothing terrestrial could occur without celestial influence. While the four elements, themselves of heavenly origin, conferred form and constitution on living beings and were consistent, a further vivifying quality was supplied by the fifth essence, the spirit, which was thought to unify the parts into a single, organic whole; cause generation and growth; and provide for sensation and movement.

Instances of the astral body appearing sometimes in the guise of the spiritual body (more acceptable to orthodoxy) occur in medical treatises and often in discussion of the immaterial cause of disease, as in Jean Fernel's *De abditis rerum causis* (1548). Spirit, conceived as an invisible constituent of the human being, was considered the medium that tied together the body and the soul. It distributed life throughout the body, initiated movement, and conducted information gathered by the senses to the captain of the body, the soul. For Paracelsus, the whole world was pervaded by spirit in continual movement, the source of the dynamic power inhering in matter. This goes some way to explain why Paracelsus was not much interested in anatomy, which was experiencing something of a vogue in his lifetime. He sought the hidden reality behind rigid structures—and a reality more authentic than what can be seen or felt was that of instinct, spirit, and life. Spirit solidified into matter and was resolved again into spirit. By means of separation and sublimation, the alchemist reverses the processes of construction back to spirit.

There was no doubt in Paracelsus's mind that there was a connection between all living things and the universe by means of dynamic forces moving continually between the celestial and terrestrial worlds. Fire and life depend upon air: "[S]ince fire cannot burn without the presence of air, one may say of the element of fire that it is of itself nothing other than a body to the soul, or perhaps a house in which the soul of man lives. Therefore fire is the true man about which our whole philosophy is concerned."[11] Respiration and combustion—similar processes in Paracelsus's mind, because fire and air are essential components in both—have mundane and celestial counterparts.

> Now the first thing we need to know is that air and fire are not palpable *corpora*, but they are perceptible and visible. And what is true in the heavens is also true in the human being: such *corpora* [as these are what] have the diseases. And just as the sun can either harm or help, so the *corpora* of the body are assaulted as the earth is by the sun. The heart is not the sun, nor the brain the moon, and so on. For the heart, the brain, etc., cohere with the sphere of the other elements. And [yet] just as the heavens operate upon them, so also upon the human being,

understood as a *corpus*. What could you possibly expect to treat without this foundation [of medicine]? Would you seek the diseases [in] physical [form], which are not physical and have no *corpora*? . . . You should also know that there is one part of the diseases of the firmament that act within the other part [of the cosmic scheme]. This simply means that you should know that earth and water never become afflicted or infirm unless the cause comes from the upper firmament. For if they become corrupt, they have been corrupted by air and the heavens.[12]

Describing the nature of diseases, Paracelsus identifies five sources of disease, derived from Hippocrates, which emanate from active principles (*entia*) and "govern our bodies and do violence to them":

The stars have a force and efficiency that has power over our body, so that it must always be ready to serve them. This virtue of the stars is called *ens astrorum*, and it is the first *ens* to which we are subjected. The second power that governs us and that inflicts diseases upon us is *ens veneni*, the influence of poison. Even if the stars are sound and have done no injury to the subtle body in us, this *ens* can destroy us; therein we are subject to it and cannot defend ourselves against it. The third *ens* is a power that injures and weakens our body even when the two other influences are beneficent; it is called *ens naturale*, the natural constitution. If it goes astray or disintegrates, our body becomes sick. From this many other diseases, indeed all diseases can arise, even if the other *entia* are sound. The fourth *ens*, the *ens spirituale*—the spiritual entity—can destroy our bodies and bring various diseases upon us. And even if all four *entia* are propitious to us and are sound, yet the fifth *ens*, the *ens Dei*, can make our bodies sick. Therefore none of the *entia* deserves as much attention as this last one; for by it one can recognize the nature of all other diseases. [. . .] Note moreover, that the various diseases do not come from one cause, but from five.[13]

Paracelsus understood that air was a starry emanation endowed with a vital property of celestial fire, which he called an aerial nitre or saltpeter.[14] Astral emanations were the means whereby the celestial ideogram could be imprinted on earthly things and read as "signatures" by the physician. In the mesocosm of the imagination, the spirit-led physician could attract and utilize these dynamic forces to produce a cure in a patient or to transmute a substance.

In his later career, from the 1530s onward, Paracelsus turned to natural magic within his comprehensive philosophy of nature. Like Marsilio Ficino (1433–1499), he believed that good magic turned on the power to draw down celestial influences, and, because the essences of everything were located in the stars, the alchemist must begin his transmutation in alignment with celestial forces. In *Erklerung der ganzen astronomei* [Explanation of All Astronomy] (ca. 1536), Paracelsus includes among the abilities of the astrologer the *artes incertae*—the arts of the imagination—that came to have a special role in his thinking. The essence of one thing could be connected to the essence of another by means of the projection of the imagination into their astral states, thus establishing an active sympathy between the two.

Paracelsus derived his notion of the astral body directly from his theory of the macrocosm and the microcosm. Paracelsus conceived of all creation as having two parts: a visible elemental (material) part and an invisible super-elemental (astral) part. The human being, the microcosm, likewise possesses an elemental body and an astral body (*corpus sidereum*). The world of matter serves the body, and the world of action and power serves the spirit because it is able to communicate with the astral part of the macrocosm. In his *Astronomia Magna or the Whole Philosophia Sagax of the Great and Little World* (1529–30), he wrote:

Man has two bodies: one from the earth, the second from the stars, and thus they are easily distinguishable. The elemental, material body goes to the grave along with its essence; the sidereal, subtle body dissolves gradually and goes back to its source, but the spirit of God in us, which is like His image, returns to Him whose image it is. Thus each part dies in that medium from which it has been created, and finds rest accordingly.

The world machine is made of two parts—one tangible and perceptible, the other invisible and imperceptible. The tangible part is the body, the invisible is the stars. The tangible part is in turn composed of three parts—Sulphur, Mercury, and Salt; the invisible also consists of three parts—feeling, wisdom, and art. The two parts together constitute life . . . all creatures in the world are made thus; and all creatures are divided into these two parts, the sensible and the insensible. The sensible is twofold, the rational and irrational but both relate to the animal nature.

The light of Nature in man comes from the stars and his flesh and blood come from material elements. Thus two influences operate in man. The first is the heavenly light in natural wisdom, art and reason. . . . The second influence emanates from matter and includes concupiscence, eating, drinking and everything that relates to the flesh and blood.[15]

The terms *astral* and *heavenly* occur frequently in Paracelsus's account of correspondences between the macrocosm and the microcosm. He constantly invokes the two sides of creation: visible and invisible, elemental and celestial, carnal and spiritual. Yet Paracelsus appeared to break with medieval astrology by asserting the limitation of astral powers. According to him, they determine neither a human being's nature, nor his behavior, nor even the span of his life. The visible stars had no causal influence. Rather, their power lay in the heavenly coordination and correspondences at work among objects and phenomena. Paracelsus also noted a correspondence between each planet and a particular seat of disease. He maintained that the stars could help direct the virtues of remedies to the diseased organ in the body, and that the physician should thus know how to achieve a concordance between the planet and the remedial herb.[16]

A theory of matter proposing a dynamic, active relationship between humans and nature informs all Paracelsus's work. For him, the imagination was not just a human faculty, but also a fundamental cosmic power of creation that was crucially connected to will and desire. Through an understanding of the *semina,* or intelligences, in matter and in himself, together with the principles denoted by his triad of sulphur, salt, and mercury, the alchemist could equally influence the corresponding intelligences of natural and spiritual elements in order to perfect what nature had left in an imperfect state.[17]

> Therefore you should know that the perfect Imagination coming from the Astral, issues from the Soul, wherein all Astra lie occult, and the Soul, Faith and Imagination, are three things to count, for the names are different, but they have equal force and strength, for one comes from the other, and I cannot compare it otherwise than with the Divine Trinity. For through the Soul we come to God, through Faith to Christ and through the Imagination to the Holy Spirit. Therefore also is to these three, even as to the holy Trinity, nothing impossible.[18]

The formation of bodies in general is comparable to the condensation of an invisible smoke, but it is not altogether converted into body, for there remains in it something eternal: the soul. Thus we have both an elemental (physical) body and a super-elemental (astral) body (*corpus sidereum*). Though the physical body is concerned solely with carnal desires, the astral body enables human communication with the super-elemental world of the *astra,* meaning the virtues, qualities, and specificity of all natural objects.

The Archeus

For Paracelsus, Creation was the result of an alchemical process, so that an understanding of alchemy was, as far as he was concerned, the only basis for practicing medicine. He predicted a revolution that was to occur shortly in medicine, when the knowledge derived from alchemy and spagyrics, of the arcana and the quintessence, would in future distinguish the doctor-magus from the followers of those he ironically terms "Father *Galen* and Father *Avicenna*": "There will be [*medici*] geo-

mantici. There will be *adepti.* There will be *archei.* There will be *spagyrici.* They will possess the *quintum esse.* They will possess the *arcana.* They will possess the *mysteria.* They will possess the *tinctura.*[19]

The knowledge of alchemy extended into all things. The living body was an alchemical retort endowed with life forces, *archei,* that acted as internal alchemists. Each organ had its own alchemist or archeus that separated from the blood the material required by the organ; thus Paracelsus's understanding of metabolism was alchemical. The chief alchemist of the body was in the stomach, where nutrients were separated from food, and poison was safely removed. But more than this, the archeus was an energy that surrounded and penetrated all things. As far as Paracelsus was concerned, there was an archeus in the patient and in the remedy, but alchemy was the external means of liberating the healing archeus from the herb. In *Paragranum,* Paracelsus finds in the alchemical work a similar process of "digestion" by which the astral virtues in medication can be separated out, revealing the arcana, which can be directed against disease.[20] Sir Thomas Browne agreed that the archeus was a spiritual agency at work not just in the assimilation of food, but also in a shared participation in the *anima mundi* so that, in an echo of the Eucharist, where participants become one with the body of Christ, the food "by one act of the soul may be converted into the body of the living, and enjoy one common soul."[21]

The Belgian chemist, Jan Baptista van Helmont (1582–1644), took up Paracelsus's concept of *workman,* as both men termed the archeus. For van Helmont, the archeus lay deep within living organisms and was responsible for their specificity, growth, and development, and their ability to transmute (metabolize). According to the American alchemist George Starkey (1628–1665), also known under the pseudonym Eirenaeus Philalethes, the archeus of disease was an irritant to the archeus residing in the body. This disease archeus was something that had to be pacified by treatment in order to restore the innate archeus to health, mirroring the ancient idea of pleasing the gods in the temples of Asclepius, from which we derive the word *placebo.* From Paracelsus and van Helmont, the Swedish scientist Emanuel Swedenborg (1688–1772) derived and developed the notion of the archeus as a natural creative power flowing from the primal substance of nature into a life principle that acted in everything. This was an idea drawn from mystical philosophy: the archeus was a creative, directive, dynamic force. Van Helmont defined it as meaning "a living aura, protector and sustainer of all things" (*aura vitalis, productor et sustentator omnium rerum*),[22] which resided in the blood or *spiritus vitalis*, called by Swedenborg the *fluidum spirituosum:* "There is a certain formative substance [*Substantia*] or force [*Vis formatrix*], that draw the thread from the first living point, and afterwards continues it to the last point of life. This is called by some the plastic force [*Vis plastica*], and the *Archeus;* by others, simply nature in action."[23]

If Paracelsus's interpretation of medicine, alchemy, theology, and cosmology was idiosyncratic, then his synthesis of them was even more so. There were several fronts on which his opponents could attack him, and he was widely misunderstood by both his supporters and his critics. His was a personal revelation based on his understanding of Hermetic and Neoplatonic philosophy, his alchemical and medical knowledge gleaned from all manner of excurricular sources, his intuition, his acute observations of the body both in sickness and in health, his insight into the workings of nature, and his imagination. This "personal wisdom"[24] is that of the magus still working with concepts that are more symbolic than chemical and more religious than scientific, and with a medical doctrine that still upheld a spiritual estimate of the human being, the microcosm.

For Paracelsus, the human world and the cosmos were indissolubly linked: "[H]eaven is man, and man is heaven."[25] Therefore, Paracelsus reasoned that the human being had to be treated with medicines that were also "spiritualized." A concept fundamental to Paracelsus is the "pneumatisation" of matter.[26]

In a way unique to his time, Paracelsus perceived that change and movement underlie the appearances of fixity, solidity, and passivity. Creation was in a continuous state of becoming as a result of the perpetual movement of the spirit. All nature was in a dynamic state of change: matter was continually solidified out of spirit, a process that could be reversed in alchemy by the spiritual motive power of elements and principles. The interaction and interpenetration of celestial and terrestrial spheres represented the Hermetic relationship between the macrocosm and the microcosm. The human world was continually in communication with celestial forces, "for the sun and the moon and all planets, as well as all the stars and the whole chaos are in man."[27] The movement was top down, coming from beyond stars and mediated in some way by the stars. But there was also a movement that was bottom up, a complementary activity arising from the nature of matter itself, which contains particles of a world soul continually seeking a return to the world of nonbeing. Almost a hundred and fifty years later, Sir Isaac Newton (1642–1727) proposed in his *Third Law of Motion* that to every action there is an equal and opposite reaction. He also intuited some power in living things that partakes of the universal life, and that in a dynamic medium, there is a reciprocal movement between matter and the incorporeal soul.

> Life and will are active Principles by wch [sic] we move our bodies, and thence arise other laws of motion unknown to us. And since all matter duly formed is attended with signes of life & all things are framed with perfect art & wisdom & Nature does nothing in vain: if there be an universal life and all space be the sensorium of a thinking being who by immediate presence perceives their pictures in the brain, the laws of motion arising from life or will may be on universal extent.[28]

In this century, science has begun to discover that nature is indeed surprisingly active, and that matter, once thought of as fixed, is also ambiguous and changeable. Developments in quantum mechanics, chaos mathematics, entanglement theory, and complexity science now acknowledge the dynamism inherently residing in matter. As Richard Gerber states in his book, *Vibrational Medicine,* "energy and matter are dual expressions of the same universal substance. That universal substance is a primal energy or vibration of which we are all composed."[29]

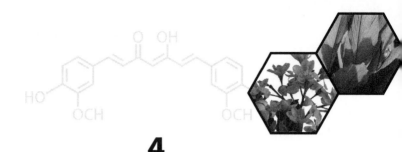

4

The Vital Force

Samuel Hahnemann
and Homeopathy

Like Paracelsus, Samuel Hahnemann was an uncompromising medical doctor who rejected the medical orthodoxy of his time and sought the wisdom of earlier traditions and the proof of experience. Hahnemann developed the similimum theory of "like curing like" and gave it a logical framework and rationale. How much he knew about alchemy is still unclear, but his idea of the vital force, the recuperative powers of the human body, the immateriality of disease, and the use of spiritlike energy medicines give him a special place in this book.

Christian Samuel Hahnemann (1755–1833) was born in Meissen, an ancient town founded in 920 on the River Elbe in Saxony by King Henry the Fowler. Hahnemann's grandfather, father, and uncle were all porcelain painters at the famous factory founded in 1710. The family background was Pietist, and he was educated at St. Afra's, the *Fürstenschule*—the prince's school—one of the premier Pietist and classical schools in Germany, which included Lessing among its distinguished alumni. Hahnemann's father used to force the young Samuel to think by setting him a problem and leaving him shut in a room by himself until he had come up with the answer. In later life, Hahnemann took as his motto *Aude sapere:* Dare to know.

A precocious linguist, the twelve-year-old Hahnemann assisted at the school by teaching the younger pupils Greek. Hahnemann went on to study medicine at Leipzig and then in Vienna, probably the finest medical school in Europe at that time. He left without a degree and later, in 1779, qualified at Erlangen. In the interval he worked as physician and librarian to Baron Samuel von Bruckenthal, governor of Transylvania, at his residence in Hermannstadt (now Sibiu, Romania). Bruckenthal was president of the Freemason's Lodge of St. Andreas zu den drei Seeblättern, and in 1777, Hahnemann was admitted to the lodge at the age of twenty-two. These contacts furnished Hahnemann with extensive access to esoteric literature on alchemy, theosophy, Rosicrucianism, and Freemasonry.

Within eight years of qualifying as a doctor, Hahnemann had become so appalled by the medical practices of his time that he stopped practicing, and from 1782 to 1796 he earned his living as a translator. Making full use of his prodigious linguistic skills, he translated texts on medicine, philosophy, art, and literature from French, Italian, English, Greek, Latin, and Hebrew. As a brilliant chemist, he perfected a preparation for soluble mercury and published a four-volume *Apothecaries' Lexicon* (1793).

The first statement of his new paradigm—"Experiment on a New Principle of Discovering the Curative Powers of the Drug Substances," in which he outlines the conduct of provings and the concept of *similar suffering* (*similia similibus curentur*)—was published in Christoph Hufeland's *Journal der praktischen Arzneikunde* in 1796, the same year that Hufeland published his *Art of Prolonging Life,* which outlined the dietary method of macrobiotics.

The full statement of Hahnemann's new medical system was *The Organon of Rational Medicine* (1810), which he continued to revise. There were six editions, the last being published posthumously in 1922. Hahnemann's new medical paradigm was so far-reaching that even he could not have understood its full import. His friend and publisher, Christoph Hufeland, recognized that if homeopathy was proved correct, major scientific dogmas would be called into question. This uncomfortable relationship to conventional thinking was present at the inception of homeopathy, and thus it has remained for two hundred years. Homeopathy is still on the fringes of conventional science. Yet Hahnemann's thought was eccentric even with respect to the mainstream of German Romantic natural science (*Naturphilosophie*) in the period 1795–1820—precisely on account of his determined stand for empiricism. In this respect, his medical thought tended to reflect the late Enlightenment, with its old-style rationalism tempered by a quickening interest in creativity, originality, and particularity, which found expression in Pre-Romanticism in the period of his youth and early medical career from 1765–1785. These currents, typified by the political critique of the young "geniuses" of the *Sturm and Drang*, would find a later efflorescence in the Romantic nationalism that attended the years of French dominance and German liberation between 1806 and 1813, the very years when Hahnemann began to articulate his medical system based on metaphors of energy, reaction, and recovery.[1]

Hahnemann's roots in Pietism, the mysticism of Jacob Boehme, and the background of Enlightenment eclecticism, with its interests in alchemy and Freemasonry, place him firmly within the compass of *Naturphilosophie*. Though he deplored and tried to distance himself from what he regarded as "the futility of transcendental speculation,"[2] Hahnemann could not ignore the metaphysical implications of his theories. The science of homeopathy takes wholly for granted the reality of what lies beyond the reach of the human senses, even beyond senses sharpened by the microscope. With its concept of a spiritlike vital force; its theory of the dynamic, spiritlike nature of disease; and its highly potentized spiritlike medicines, homeopathy defies materialist notions of the body and of the disease.

Immateriality of Disease

Hahnemann distinguished between two kinds of disease: those with a simple explanation, such as a foreign body, and those that are unknowable. To him, disease belonged to "the secrets of nature no created mind can penetrate."[3] Disease was the last unknowable mystery: Its cause could not be known "since it is not discernible and is not to be found. Since most diseases (indeed the vast majority of them) are of a dynamic spirit-like origin and of dynamic spirit-like nature, their cause is not discernible to the senses."[4]

> When a person falls ill, it is initially only this spirit-like, autonomic life force (life principle), everywhere present in the organism, that is mistuned through the dynamic influence of a morbific agent inimical to life. Only the life principle, mistuned to such abnormality can impart to the organism the adverse sensations and induce in the organism the irregular functions that we call disease. The life principle is a power-*Wesen* invisible in itself, only discernible by its effect on the organism. [. . .] The morbid mistunement of the life principle makes itself discernible by disease symptoms; in no other way can it make itself known. [*Organon* §11]
>
> Therefore disease (excluding surgical cases) is not what allopaths believe it to be. Disease is not to be considered as an inwardly hidden *Wesen* separate from the living whole, from the organism and its enlivening *dynamis*, even if it is thought to be very subtle. Such an absurdity could only arise in brains of a materialist stamp. It is this absurdity that has . . . fashioned [medicine] into a truly calamitous art. [*Organon* §13][5]

This view of disease dispenses with the neat linear model of cause and effect, which blames bacteria for disease. Far from being the cause, Hahnemann considers bacteria to be merely the scavengers of disease. For him, illness is something more spiritual and dynamic that affects the organism from within, an alteration arising at some deep level of the psyche. Illness signals that the person is incomplete and their vital force is not in order or harmony. Unless there is a return to health, symptoms will continue to erode the freedom of the patient. Illness disturbs patterns of behavior in order to force a change. If we are alert to illness and allow ourselves to be disturbed by it, we can come to see its corrective powers. As the American homeopath Kent argued, "no disease can impose itself upon the physical body through its ultimate forms." The disease must come from the higher dynamic plane of the soul. Thus "the soul adapts the human body to all its purposes, the higher purposes of its being."[6] The disease, originating in the higher plane, descends to the corporeal plane, where it creates disturbance at the functional level. The disease becomes embodied, which in turn reverses the message and sends it back into the sphere of consciousness, where, if correctly understood, it can bring about the will to change. To complete the cure, argues Twentyman, "healing must involve a change in consciousness as well as a change in somatic symptoms. Something unconscious or forgotten must be recalled or something allowed to sink into forgetfulness."[7]

For this reason, "all curable maladies have signs and symptoms to make themselves known."[8] If disease manifests itself in order to bring about change in a corresponding inner process, it is itself homeopathic, curing like with like, and as the patient recovers, he or she moves into a higher plane of being, where the lower potency remedy no longer touches him. "When a patient has been carried up through a series of potencies he will often remain unaffected by that remedy in a lower realm of potency."[9]

The Influence of Swedenborgianism on Homeopathy

Hahnemann's new medical system exemplified German Romantic medicine in its emphasis on subtle, inner energies; its vision of the human being, health, and disease as a theatre of intangible metaphysical forces operating in a wider cosmos of fundamental principles that animate, enliven, and maintain the universe of responsive beings in a living world. Hahnemann's anthropology and cosmology owe a strong debt to Pietistic notions of individuality within a meaningful, beneficent, and purposeful universe. There are also indications that such ideas, germane to Pietism and its legacy to the late Enlightenment, also partook of Boehmean mysticism, which had continued to flow through Pietistic thought, and the eclectic currents of the Enlightenment.

To this mixture, Hahnemann's greatest interpreter, the American-born James Tyler Kent (1849–1916), added Swedenborgianism, and this influence has been so complete and profound that now "it may not be possible to return directly to Hahnemann."[10] Born in Sweden, Emanuel Swedenborg (1688–1772), a brilliant polymath, made significant contributions to mining, mathematics, navigation, and anatomy. In 1743–1744, mystical experiences led to the opening of his spirit vision, and he subsequently devoted his life to writing a revelatory theology. Though he founded no sect himself, his followers began a Church of the New Jerusalem in 1787, which now has branches throughout the world. Hahnemann himself had acknowledged the supremacy of the animating spirit—the vital force—within the living organism. Like Emanuel Swedenborg, Hahnemann recognized the spiritual nature of humans and the body as the servant of that spirit. But, although Hahnemann was keenly interested in psychological states, in his original writings he did not emphasize mental and emotional symptoms over physical ones. Yet Kent took the view that the medicine must be directed not to the body itself, but toward healing the split between the will and understanding, for, he argues: "[M]an consists in what he thinks and what he loves and there is nothing else in man [. . .] all medicines operate upon the will and understanding first."[11]

What Kent contributed to homeopathy was the Swedenborgian idea of the inner and outer human, from which he developed the idea of internals and externals and the gradations between them—a series of degrees from the divine (sublime) to the ultimate (matter), with the result that *ultimates* became a widely used term for manifested illness. With Kent, homeopathic prescribing gave precedence to the mental and emotional symptoms as being finer and closer to the will and understanding. And indeed, it is now well known that cells are acted upon by hormones and peptides, which are directly influenced by our emotions.

A natural result of his view of the internal economy of the human being was that Kent came to prefer high potencies over lower ones. Hahnemann had mostly used 30C. (See page 67 for an explanation of C.) Higher potencies, by being further removed from the world of matter, acted more powerfully on the vital force, or *simple substance,* than lower ones. What appealed most to Kent, as an adherent to Swedenborgianism, was precisely the immateriality of the medicines, and he extended this into ever-higher potencies, up to 1M (See page 67 for an explanation of M) and beyond. Higher potencies mirrored his belief in the spiritual nature of human beings, and Kent concluded that the ability to affect the human will and understanding was the special province of homeopathic remedies.

What Kent did not know, because the sixth edition of the *Organon* was not published until after his lifetime, was that Hahnemann himself was still experimenting with potency until the very end of his career, and he too was increasingly moving away from materiality into LM dilutions (See page 68 for an explanation of LM). The similarity of their views is possibly due to their drawing upon the same sources of inspiration, from Paracelsus and Boehme to Jan Baptista van Helmont and Henry More, whom Swedenborg frequently quoted.[12] Kent reorganized the homeopathic *Repertory* to mirror the Swedenborgian principle of "from above to below," reflecting the descent from the divine being through decreasing degrees of fineness to the material level. For Kent, the material human body is not the true being, which is truly interior and subjective, enlivened by the will and the mind:

> The man wills and understands; the cadaver does not will and does not understand; then that which takes its departure is that which knows and wills. It is *that* which can be changed and is prior to the body. The combination of these two, the will and the understanding constitute man [. . .] man *is* the will and the understanding and the house which he lives in is his body.[13]

Potency

Homeopathic remedies are prepared by a process of dilution and succussion. A substance, such as an herb, is made into a tincture by steeping it in alcohol or, in the case of a mineral substance, is triturated* with sugar of milk until it can be dissolved. Then 1 drop of tincture is added to 10 parts water and is succussed vigorously (by banging it hard if prepared by hand, or by shaking it with a machine). One drop is then taken and diluted with 10 parts water, and the result is again succussed. This is the decimal potency scale, usually denoted as X. There is also a centesimal scale in which one 1 drop is diluted with 100 parts of water, and the result is succussed, diluted, and succussed repeatedly. After 5 dilutions this will be $1:10^{10}$. This potency is denoted by C, as in 6C or 30C (i.e., 6 dilutions in 100 parts of water each time, or 30 times the same). The most commonly prescribed potencies are 6C and 30C. The medicating potency is usually delivered on lactose tablets or sucrose pills for ease of transport and treatment. After twelve dilutions and succussions on the centesimal scale ($12C = 1:10^{23}$), there will not be a single molecule of the original substance present, according to Avogadro's Law.

There is a millesimal dilution scale, denoted by M, as in 1M, 10M, and 50M. Paradoxically, but in keeping with Kent's philosophy, the higher potency remedies are often the more effective, though this does depend upon the condition being treated. Homeopathy has often been ridiculed for its extreme dilution: how can a remedy that contains not one molecule of the original substance have any effect? Yet critics tend to overlook the shock imparted to the remedy by succussion. This shock is thought to imprint the subtle energetic qualities of the substance used and to amplify the vibrational signature of the therapeutic pattern.

---

*Trituration is a method of remedy preparation in which an insoluble medicinal substance is reduced by grinding with a carrier such as sugar of milk. Sugar of milk is lactose.

Hahnemann was quite aware that, at his preferred potency of 30C, his homeopathic remedies were unlikely to have a molecular presence of the original substance, which is why he termed them "spirit-like." The nonmateriality of the remedy has made it possible to use in the homeopathic armamentarium what would otherwise be poisons, such as arsenic, belladonna, and deadly snake venoms (e.g., cobra, rattlesnake, and lachesis [bushmaster]). The word *pharmacy* means both "remedy" and "poison." As Paracelsus claimed, the difference between them is in the dose. At the end of his career, Hahnemann moved toward the LM potency, also known as Q, which is the quinquaginta-millesimal dilution scale. Hahnemann describes this scale in paragraphs 246–48, 270, 271, and 278 of the sixth edition of *The Organon*.

Hahnemann was concerned with the vital force of the living being at the innermost part of the patient that was not only invisible, but also immortal. He called this the *vital force* or *life-sustaining power,* and it is the counterpart to Swedenborg's *life spirit, life fluid,* or *spiritual fluid* (*fluidum spirituosum*). James Tyler Kent called the vital force *simple substance* and the "vice-regent of the soul."[14]

The Principles of Homeopathy

For Hahnemann, there was no contradiction between his emphasis on empiricism and the fact that his highly potentized medicines were beyond material substance. It was sufficient that clearly observable effects on healthy experimenters, when they "proved" the medicines, and on patients in recovery showed that they worked. This mixture of empiricism in the realm of the "spirit-like" was possibly the outcome of Hahnemann's time and place. Though he built with old materials, such as the law of similars adopted from Hippocates and Paracelsus, he brought forth a complete, organized, and coherent system of unchanging principles. Whereas conventional medicine frequently changes its methods with regard to drugs or surgical intervention, homeopathy is founded upon principles based upon the meticulous observation of the human body both in sickness and in health.

These principles consist of the proposition that there is a vital force, that susceptibility is an agent both in illness and in its cure, that like cures like, and that "provings" determine the likeness of curative ability.*

Proving

To establish the curative powers of a remedy, it is necessary to *prove* them. This is done by giving a group of volunteers a small dose of the substance or remedy to be proved. Hahnemann's Provers Union of family and friends usually knew what they were taking, but Kent recognized the importance of blind testing, and modern provings are carried out as random, double-blind tests, with some provers being given the remedy and other provers given placebos, or tablets of inert sugar of milk. Before taking anything, provers first make notes over several weeks of any symptoms, indispositions, or discomforts they habitually experience. After taking the remedy, they make notes of any changes in their state, and these are attributed to the therapeutic power of the substance, which cures in the sick the same symptoms it produces in the healthy.

Beginning with Peruvian bark, which was used to treat malaria, Hahnemann proved some hundred substances on himself and claimed that the process strengthened his constitution. Self-provings had already been conducted by Conrad Gesner (1516–1565), Giorgio Baglivi (1660–1742), Thomas Sydenham (1624–1689), and Friedrich Hoffman (1660–1742). Albrecht von Haller described the desirability of physicians testing medicines on themselves in his *Pharmacopeia* (Basel, 1771), which Hahnemann quotes with approval. Provings were frequently undertaken by Franz Anton Mesmer's friend Anton Störck (1731–1803) at the Vienna Medical School.

---

*The fundamental Hippocratic principle that "like cures like" had also been articulated by Georg Ernst Stahl in his *Commentatio de arthritide tam tartarea, quam scorbutica, seu podagra et scorbuto* [A Treatise on Diseases of the Joint, both Hellish and Scurvy-like: Gout and Scurvy], 1738.[15]

Vital Force

The central tenet of homeopathy is the vital force. Medical students typically spend their first weeks of instruction on the corpse, in all its grim gradations of decay. Once dissection and anatomy has familiarized them with the structure of the body as it is in death, they are brought into the wards, where they encounter the living. Here, students find an important difference between the living and the dead, a difference so obvious and striking as to pass without comment. Here, even in the sick, is the mysterious, magical, and mystical quality of aliveness that marks the living from the dead. In these patients, the vital force still flows, the *dynamis* (see below) is dramatically at work, the animating principle is still in command. Here too, probably unknowingly, students find themselves at the parting of the ways between conventional and complementary medicine and the very different estimates of the two regarding life, energy, health, and disease. In the wards, they find revealed all the ravages that disease can wreak, and pathology then becomes a major part of their training and the basis of their practice.

Conventional medical science knows a great deal about the numerous ways in which the body deteriorates in disease, but it does not have a fully developed theory of the vital force and the dynamis that keeps a person well. Many people, observing living beings, would take as self-evident the proposition that the life force exists. Yet within the medical profession, there is a determined and vocal group whose position is that "there is no evidence whatsoever for a life force."[16]

Dynamis

Related to the vital force is the idea that every part is enlivened by its own dynamic power, so that "Vital force and Soul are in the cell as well as in the body. The same thing rules the remedy and, stripped of its grossness and placed upon the tongue, it will be taken into the economy instantly."[17]

Dynamis is what Hahnemann called the *immaterial vital principle,* and it obviously has parallels with Paracelsus's ideas of the archeus.

For James Tyler Kent it was an energy "endowed with formative intelligence" (*vis formatrix*) which maintains order and harmony in the universe no less than in the human body. "The body does not move, think, or act unless it has its interior degrees of immaterial substance which acts upon the economy in the most beautiful manner."[18] The energy flows and, because it flows, it is subject to change; it can flow in order or in disorder. It is an energy and a force, a dynamis possessing power.[19] It is the dynamis that lends the body its seemingly miraculous powers of self-regulation and recovery, when the dynamis in the remedy is matched to the dynamis of the disease. It works though a synergy of dynamis and the physical structure. In his book, *Vibrational Medicine*, Richard Gerber suggests that each cell in a living body is a "hologram" containing the energetic imprint of the whole:

> All organisms are dependent upon a subtle vital force which creates synergism via a unique structural organisation of molecular components. Because of this synergism, the living whole is greater than the sum of its parts. The vital force creates order in living systems and constantly rebuilds and renews its cellular vehicle of expression.[20]

Susceptibility

The body has a powerful sense of its own self, and like any sovereign country, it patrols its borders. Like a vast army composed of many ranks and forces, the immune system mobilizes continually against invasion. A class of proteins known as fibroblast growth factor (FGF), fibroblasts, and connective tissue become an army at the ready, standing by to respond to signals from molecules to repair wounds, fractures, and pathological change.

Contrary to the position of orthodox medicine is the holistic view that the signs and symptoms of disease are not caused by external agents, but rather come about through the body's attempt to maintain its own homeostasis. Samuel Hahnemann reasoned that if the signs and symptoms of disease are not actually disease, the disease must be something else, something altogether less tangible. The cause of illness may be lowered immunity, but what cause can be found for that? There seems to be another aspect to immunity, which is the link between the mind and the body. This more subtle form of energy, which regulates our state of health and vitality, is the complex interplay between nutritional health, hygiene, and emotional well-being or psychic health.

When the Nereid Thetis dipped Achilles into the River Styx in order to make him invulnerable, she held him by the heel and so left a hole or weak point in his immunity. Paris later killed Achilles by sending a poisoned arrow into his heel. The Greek myth of Achilles has become a byword for a tragic flaw and immune failure. It demonstrates an idea of immunity to which Paracelsus adhered: the notion of holes in the immune system through which invaders can pass, and these are as much breaches in our psychic defenses as physical ones. It is a negative or minus condition of being, a state of lowered resistance that we recognize and call *susceptibility.*

The cell's regulating DNA is acted on by chemical reactions. This is enough for the conventional scientist—but it has also been clinically demonstrated that cells appear to have some form of intelligence that directs their function, and that the mind can communicate with cells and thus influence their activity and DNA. In 1974, Robert Ader found that the central nervous system and the immune system are in constant communication.* Since then, evidence for the clinical importance of emotions has been mounting, giving rise to a new branch of medical science—*psychoneuroimmunology* (PNI)—and making psychotherapy one of the fastest growing therapies.

The chemical messengers that operate most extensively between brain and the immune system are most dense in the neural areas that

---

*Robert Ader is currently simultaneously professor of medicine, professor of psychiatry, and professor of clinical and social psychology at the University of Rochester, Rochester, N.Y.

respond to emotion, which we experience both as a state of agitation in the mind and also a manifestation in the physical body. If cells can receive messages directly from the mind, emotions are literally embodied at the cellular level, and we are made ill not by circumstance alone, but also by ourselves. Joyful white blood cells possess powerful immune competence; unhappy, stressed, angry, or despairing cells cannot function with full vigor, and the immune system is thereby compromised. It has been well demonstrated that hypnosis and meditation produce physical results such as anesthetization. Invading cells can also be influenced by the mind; a change in attitude can cause illnesses to remit, and visualization techniques have been found to shrink cancers measurably. This fact should not surprise us; if the mind has played a part in the onset of a condition, it is likely to play a part in its retreat.

Spiritual healing, shown in dramatic and extreme acceleration of the processes of organic repair and with physical restoration accompanied by spiritual growth, is sufficiently well-attested throughout the world to point to an immaterial component of illness. That immaterial component manifests itself through our susceptibility. Disease is a distortion of the hidden genatrix of life. Disease is transferred to the physical body and makes itself known through our susceptibility, which then takes up an infectious agent or disease manifestation. Thus James Tyler Kent can claim that there are no diseases, only sick people, and the sick person will be made sick under every circumstance. If there is a purpose to illness, our susceptibility will, like a vacuum, draw the disease to itself, and will take up as much of the morbific agent as it requires. Like the organism, susceptibility has an appetite, and knows how much sickness it needs. The individual's susceptibility to disease has to be satisfied in the first place by the morbific agent it attracts to itself. Homeopathy, by introducing a close match to the symptoms of sickness, can satisfy the susceptibility in such a way that it no longer needs the illness, a notion recalling Paracelsus's description of the curative remedy as the *bride* of the disease.

Whereas allopathic medicine delivers broad-spectrum drugs in a dose related to the intensity of the pathology, homeopathy matches the potency of the medicine to the degree of susceptibility of the patient, with the intention of modifying it. Stuart Close claims that "this power to *modify susceptibility* is the basis of the art of the physician . . . since cure consists simply in satisfying the morbid susceptibility of the organism and putting an end to the influx of disease-producing causes."[21] Chinese medicine also has a concept of deficient *chi* as a precursor of many illnesses. Herbs and acupuncture are used specifically to build the chi in key areas of the body and so halt the onset of illness.

The word *susceptibility* derives from the Latin *suscipere,* "to take up." It denotes our capacity to take up or receive impressions, and the word applies as much to emotional impressions as physical ones. According to Close, "susceptibility is one of the fundamental attributes of life. Upon it depends all functioning, all vital processes, physiological and pathological."[22]

Susceptibility, whether of mind or body, is a state, and because the taking on of states "is the history of human life," to do anything to impede the ability to take on states is to align "with the forces of death and destruction."[23] It is good ecology to preserve the susceptibility of the organism and its power to react to stimuli, because without susceptibility, there can be no illness, no cure, no change, no development.

Susceptibility relates not merely to immune failure, but also to attraction and desire, hunger and need. Like the organism itself, disease has its own susceptibility, its own attraction, hunger, and need. As the patient hungers for food, the disease hungers for medicine, and what will appease it is the medicine that most closely resembles it. In homeopathic thinking, the remedies depend for their effectiveness on susceptibility—the reactiveness or impressionability of the organism. Some susceptibility will exist toward a range of medicines, but the highest degree of susceptibility is toward the nearest match, the *similimum,* or equal.

Susceptibility exists apart from disease. It is only while the symptoms of the disease are active that the medicines are homeopathic. Once the disease has been satisfied, there is a change of state, and the medicine ceases to act homeopathically. Instead, the susceptibility of the body takes up the medicine in a different way, and the medicines no longer act curatively but aggressively or depressively. This susceptibility is precisely what orthodox medicine fails to recognize when it dismisses as side effects the unwanted results of treatment, which account for the vast range of iatrogenic cases filling our hospitals.

Samuel Hahnemann recognized that, because of susceptibility, no substance introduced into the body can do only good and no harm whatever. In his potentized remedies, therefore, he attempted to create something as immaterial and subtle as the dynamis itself, something that would align itself with the native intelligence of the body and rely on the subtle attunement of susceptibility to perceive it and take it up. "This *dynamic* action of medicines, the vitality itself by means of which it is reflected upon the organism, is almost purely *spiritual* in its nature."[24]

The symptoms of the disease create a kind of template or matrix upon which the homeopathic medicine can be laid down, matching the configuration of the disease as closely as possible, satisfying it, and ultimately taking its place—ousting the sickness, and then fading away. Where illness is disharmony, homeopathy invites order, stimulating the vital force and engaging "the organism in the most creative and curative response of which it is capable."[25]

Illness is in our nature, and so is the potential for healing and cure. These are part of our cosmic realignment and potential for transformation. It is our susceptibility that makes this possible; without it we could learn nothing, change nothing. Susceptibility goes with our differentiation, polarity, individuation, and enlarged consciousness.

The further a living being advances in the direction of polarity—that is, of self-awareness—the more prone it becomes to illness. . . . Human beings display the most highly developed form of self-awareness known to us, and for that reason, it is we human beings who experience the tension of polarity at its strongest. In consequence, it is also on the human level that illness has its greatest significance.[26]

For this reason, susceptibility is extremely active in children, in whom the need for individualization is greatest.

Disease is the creative opportunity to escape stagnation and bring about transformation. The sick person will be made sick under every circumstance, because attention needs to be drawn to the direction in which our lives are moving, untangling emotional warping, and reorientating psychological patterns. Neither nature nor individuals can spend a long time in confrontation; ultimately there is yielding and assimilation. "It is illness that ultimately makes us heal-able. Illness is the turning-point at which unwholeness can start to be turned into wholeness."[27] Homeopathic medicine carries "the full power of the uncompensated-for spirit inside us . . . they are our only present clue to what may be a whole nether universe of matter and energy."[28]

It is the vital force, not the medicine, that brings a cure—but the medicine is a catalyst that operates dynamically through our susceptibility to promote a change of state on all levels. Susceptibility is our defining aspect, both collectively as human beings and singly as individuals. "[W]hat a man is susceptible to, such a man is, such is his quality."[29] We might perhaps add: what a man is susceptible to, such he will become; such is his opportunity.

Polarity is the energy of the universe. In the dynamic nature of life, we live with light and dark, health and sickness, life and death, and on the continuum between them. In the theatre of forces, each human heart trembles between powers seeking resolution. Susceptibility is a profound aspect of our nature; it is the fulcrum on which the polarity of life turns. Susceptibility exists because life is not static, but instead tends to growth, development, and transformation. Susceptibility is required because we are mortal, incomplete, conflict-ridden, lacking wholeness and oneness. Yet we have the capacity to yearn for immortality, completion, peace, wholeness, and unity. Susceptibility exists because human beings inhabit divided and distinguished worlds—we move between earth and heaven, the material and the transcendent—and we are divided and distinguished beings, neither wholly spiritual nor wholly sensual, but simultaneously material and immaterial. If the spiritual part of an individual is the regulative principle of the whole person, susceptibility is its chief agent, drawing to it and taking up the impressions of life, enlarging our sympathies and self-awareness in pursuit of wholeness and realization.

What has emerged from the more sensitive engagement with plants in the twentieth century, particularly with the development of Flower Remedies, is that plants have an empathetic connection with the human being. While the mind continually returns to theory, the susceptible heart opens to the world of nature and finds there a cure and nourishment for body and soul. As Paracelsus recognized, once we begin to look with "the light of nature," we become part of the unity of all life. Plants help us to become more fully ourselves. They attune us to the spiritual dimension and "help us to develop that inner great self in all of us which has the power to overcome all fears, all difficulties, all worries, all diseases."[30]

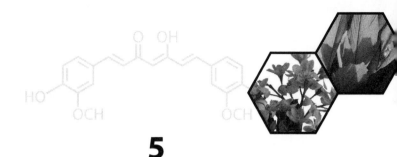

5

Neo-Paracelsian Spagyrics

The Survival of Paracelsianism in Western Esoteric Currents

The revival of Paracelsian medicine is a little-known but still-growing phenomenon within the broader realm of complementary health and intellectual and medical history. As we have seen, Paracelsus reformulated alchemy in accordance with his *Naturphilosophie,* emphasizing the two philosophical principles (Sulphur and Mercury) and adding a third, Salt. Paracelsus was chiefly interested in alchemy as a means of making medicines of great vitality and potency. He worked with metals, formulating the new science of *iatrochemistry,* and with plant alchemy called *spagyrics.*

Among the most notable scientists to have followed Paracelsus, Jan Baptista van Helmont, a capable chemist, had a lasting influence on the American George Starkey (1628–1655) and his friend Robert Boyle (1627–1691). Van Helmont first discovered gas, and he completed a number of interesting experiments. Perhaps best known is his experiment with a tree sapling: he planted a sapling after first weighing it and the dry earth. After five years, he weighed both again. Because the weight of the earth had not diminished, he concluded that the sapling's gain in growth had been due solely to the nutrients in the water that had been regularly applied to it. He did not consider that the air might also have provided some nutrients for the plant.

As a physician, van Helmont was interested in Paracelsian medical ideas. Yet it is clear that Paracelsus used only very small doses of medicines. In fact, Paracelsus had advocated "unweighable and unmeasurable doses." Over time, this important principle was ignored, and iatrochemistry became dangerous due to the zeal with which larger doses were applied.

Paracelsus left behind a large, unpublished opus. It was initially published in fragments by his followers in England, France, and Germany throughout the sixteenth century. In the 1590s, a collected edition of Paracelsus's works was published by Johannes Huser in Basel. Two major centers are associated with the transmission of Paracelsianism in the seventeenth century. In central Germany, Görlitz became an important center of Paracelsian publishing. Such figures as Bartholomaeus Scultetus, a municipal councillor and friend of Tycho Brahe and Johannes Kepler; Balthasar Walter, a Paracelsian personal physician to the prince of Anhalt and friend of Jacob Boehme; and Johann Huser, the editor of Paracelsus's works, all influenced Jacob Boehme (1575–1624) of Görlitz, the founder of modern mystical Protestant theosophy. Boehme incorporated Paracelsian and alchemical ideas in *Aurora* (1612) and his other mystical writings. Boehme's influence spread, inspiring many later theosophers in England (John Pordage and Jane Leade), Holland (Johann Georg Gichtel), America (Johannes Kelpius in Pennsylvania), and Anglo-German connections in London (Dionysius Andreas Freher).

Both Strasbourg and Basel were important stations in Paracelsus's own life. In both places, he was in close touch with circles of humanists and reformers, and these groups continued to provide a geographical setting for the later revival of alchemical and Hermetic ideas in southern Germany. Johann Valentin Andreä (1586–1654) was born into a family of eminent and distinguished Lutheran theologians and churchmen in Württemberg. His father, Johannes Andreä (1554–1601), was also interested in alchemy, and the son evidently combined these interests with his own vision of a magical, scientific, and religious reformation of the whole wide world. In Frances Yates's view, this amounted to a late efflorescence of Hermetic ideas in the context of Protestant spirituality at the very beginning of the seventeenth century. These ideas again drew on Paracelsian *Naturphilosophie*, combining theology and proto-scientific approaches to the apprehension of nature and medicine.

In southwestern Germany, Paracelsian thought led through Johann Valentin Andreä (1586–1654) to the Rosicrucian movement. With his alchemist friend Christoph Welling, Andreä traveled to Strasbourg in 1606, and together they visited Lazarus Zetzner, the publisher of Paracelsus in Strasbourg. Between 1604 and 1607, Andreä wrote his first draft of the *Chemical Wedding of Christian Rosenkreutz*, and it was finally published by Zetzner in Strasbourg in 1616. After 1609, Andreä was close to Dr. Tobias Hess, the Paracelsian enthusiast and an unorthodox tutor at Tübingen. Between 1609–1611, Andreä and his friends wrote the first version of the *Fama Fraternitatis*, the first Rosicrucian manifesto, which drew on Paracelsus as an inspiration. The Rosicrucian movement attracted many English and Continental scholars (e.g., Robert Fludd, Michael Maier, Jan Amos Comenius, Samuel Hartlib, Thomas Vaughan, Elias Ashmole).

The Rosicrucian-alchemical tradition was fostered by high-degree Masonic orders and secret societies known under the general appellation of Gold-und Rosenkreutz in eighteenth-century central Europe.[1] There was also an important overlap of this tradition with the theosophical currents prevalent among the Swabian Pietists, such as the senior prelate Friedrich Christoph Oetinger (1702–1782), who maintained an alchemical laboratory at his abbey in Murrhardt in Württemberg.

By the end of the eighteenth century, the influence of Neoplatonic and esoteric ideas resurfaced in Germany in a new current of science and medicine known as *Naturphilosophie*. Johann Wolfgang von Goethe (1749–1832) complemented his scientific work in anatomy, botany, and optics with studies in the history of alchemy and some practical experiments towards finding the elixir. The Neoplatonic philosophy of Friedrich Wilhelm Joseph von Schelling (1775–1854) inspired a young generation of Romantic scientists, including the mining engineer Friedrich von Hardenberg, better known as the Romantic poet Novalis (1772–1801); Johann Wilhelm Ritter (1776–1810); Lorenz Oken (1779–1851); and H. C. Oersted (1777–1851), all of whom were interested in polarity. The German Romantic interest in Neoplatonism and Hermetic ideas was peculiarly suited to the development of new paradigms in magnetism, electricity, and photochemistry, as well as in psychology, mesmerism, and somnambulism.

It is in this context of German Romantic natural science that we can locate the work of Samuel Hahnemann, the founder of homeopathy. His theory of the vital force demonstrates the Romantic interest in metaphysical forms of energy as well as a somewhat ambiguous debt to the thought of Paracelsus.[2]

It was at the end of the nineteenth century, in 1875, in reaction to the challenges posed by Darwinism, materialism, and secularization, that the modern Theosophical Society of Helena Blavatsky (1831–1891) was founded in New York. Taking its cue from the late-nineteenth-century interest in spiritualism and psychical research, modern Theosophy provided a portal through which many intellectuals and writers discovered the Western esoteric tradition that stretched back through the alchemists, Rosicrucians, Boehme, Paracelsus, and the scholar-magicians of the Renaissance.

Theosophy spread to Germany, England, and France. Franz Hartmann (1838–1912), a German-American theosophist, published books on Paracelsus, Jacob Boehme, and the Rosicrucians as well as on Oriental subjects. Other theosophists preferred to purge theosophy of its Oriental borrowings. Rudolf Steiner (1861–1925), general secretary of the Theosophical Society in Berlin from 1902, pioneered a new Western esoteric movement based on his work as editor of Goethe's scientific works and his rediscovery of Paracelsus and the Rosicrucian tradition. Other German theosophists drew their inspiration from the local esoteric traditions of Protestant Swabia and studied Jacob Boehme, Andreä's Rosicrucian manifestos, the theosopher F. C. Oetinger, Justinus Kerner

(1786–1862), Jakob Lorber (1800–1864), and Karl von Reichenbach (1788–1868), the discoverer of an Odic magnetic force in medicine.

The modern revival of Paracelsian and spagyric medicine—as developed by some two dozen or so pharmaceutical companies and laboratories located chiefly in Swabia, but also in other parts of Germany, America, France, Switzerland, and Australia—owe their inception to the early twentieth-century revival of interest in the Western esoteric tradition, mediated through the portal of the enduring theosophical traditions of Germany.

Neo-Paracelsian Spagyrics from the Nineteenth Century to the Present

Johann Gottfried Rademacher (1772–1850)

An important figure in the recovery of alchemical medicines was the physician Johann Gottfried Rademacher, who traced many of his ideas directly from Paracelsus and Jan Baptista van Helmont. Born in Hamm, Westphalia, on August 4, 1772, Rademacher pursued his medical studies at Jena, graduating in 1794. At Jena, he came into contact with Christoph Hufeland, who was physician to Johann Wolfgang von Goethe (1749–1832) and the founder of macrobiotics. His *naturphilosophisch* medical journal was very influential in spreading new and alternative medical approaches. Hufeland was the first to publish Hahnemann's theories, and Rademacher calls him "my old master."[3]

Rademacher began his medical practice in Goch, in Saxony, in 1794, but, like many other physicians of the time, including Samuel Hahnemann, he was unhappy about "heroic" medicine that involved extreme purges, emetics, and bloodletting. Such methods were the direct outcome of the Galenical medicine that Paracelsus and van Helmont had so despised. In eighteenth-century Europe, these methods were still widely practiced, and it was not unusual for patients to die of exsanguination as a result of repeated bloodletting.

It was his discovery of the therapeutic value of sodium nitrate (*Natrum nitricum*) that put Rademacher on the trail of the iatrochemists. He used the remedy extensively for inflammations and hemorrhages, even for pneumonia. He surmised that the remedy owed its origin to the Paracelsian iatrochemists, and so he began extensive researches into Paracelsian and van Helmontian writings on the nature of illness, methods of preparation of medicines, and therapeutics. Although Rademacher discarded most of their theories, he accepted Paracelsus's notion of specific disease entities, the minimum dose, and some organ-specific medicines. Rademacher also revived the Paracelsian doctrine of signatures in his theory of remedies and disease. Many of his medicines were made by the method of plant alchemy known as spagyrics, and he published a book in defense of the system entitled *Rechtfertigung der von den Gelehrten misskannten, verstandesrechten Erfahrungsheillehre der alten scheidekünstigen Geheimärzte* [Justification of the Empirical Medical Practice of the Old Alchemical Physicians, Misjudged by the Learned, Yet Perfectly Rational, as Verified by Twenty-five Years of Experience at the Bedside]. This work, published in 1841 and still not translated into English in its entirety, is usually called by its short German title: *Erfahrungsheillehre*. An English-language edition, much abbreviated, was published in Philadelphia by Boericke and Tafel in 1909. As the German title indicates, Rademacher based his therapeutic system on the "old spagyric physicians," demonstrating that he was prepared to go back and investigate from original sources. In this way he was able to validate much of what Paracelsus had discovered in the sixteenth century.

Like Paracelsus and his own contemporary, Samuel Hahnemann, Rademacher was an empiricist, and he followed his own independent lines of inquiry. Paracelsus was strongly influenced by the doctrine of signatures, an intimation that the herb called attention to what it could cure by resembling a part of the body. Eyebright (*Euphrasia offinalis*) is a striking example: it resembles the eye, for which it is in fact the chief medicinal herb. Rademacher rejected this notion of correspondences, and yet he noted from his own experience that some herbs did indeed appear to have a definite affinity for particular organs, whether or not they actually looked like these parts of the human body. As a result, Rademacher developed organ remedies, a therapeutic modality that came to be known as organopathy. In his practice he saw patients for whom a holistic approach was necessary, because disease arose within the organism as a whole, and he saw others whose maladies appeared to indicate an imbalance in the function of an organ. His work was based on clinical observation and experience. Yet he was also drawn to the art of medicinal alchemy, and he investigated the work of Paracelsus and the iatrochemists, as Paracelsus's followers were known.

Paracelsus had impressed upon his readers the need to understand the role of the stars in illness. Rademacher did not take up astrology, but he did notice that certain illnesses were associated with onset at a particular time. Even if the illness had become chronic and persisted for many years, it was necessary, he believed, to treat the patient with a remedy that matched the specific time when the patient first became aware of the illness.

Whereas in homeopathy it was necessary to individualize to the patient's symptoms, the affinity of certain remedies to particular organs was well known. Rademacher empirically tested the organ affinities, relating them to pathological conditions. This was his great gift to Western medicine, and his use of organ remedies was adopted by homeopathic medicine and by eclectic medicine of North America. This organ affinity is also the sphere of action where spagyric medicines are preeminent.

Initially, Rademacher's medical program was taken up eagerly, with his work appearing in six editions between 1841 and 1848. A small band of practitioners—Rademacherians, as they were dubbed—published a journal, *Zeitschrift für Erfahrungsheilkunst* [Journal for Experiential Healing]. Homeopathy, however, proved the more popular modality until the *Erfahrungsheillehre* was rediscovered by the eccentric English physician James Compton Burnett, who was intrigued by the immense success Rademacher had enjoyed in thirty years of practice right up to the end of his life.

James Compton Burnett (1840–1901)

James Compton Burnett was born in Redlynch, near Salisbury, England, but he studied medicine at the prestigious Vienna Medical School from 1865–1869, where he won a gold medal for his work in anatomy. He graduated in 1872 in Glasgow and went on to an internship at Barnhill Parochial Hospital and Asylum in Glasgow. It was during this period of internship that Burnett, disillusioned with the failures of the conventional medicine of his time, was introduced to homeopathy by Alfred Hawkes. When a child died of a fever, Burnett turned to homeopathy, but with a skeptical and inquiring mind. He relates his own empirical experiment on the children's ward at Glasgow:

> Feverish colds and chills were common enough just then, moreover, a ward where children thus taken ill were put till their diseases had declared themselves, and they were drafted off to the various wards, for that purpose provided, with pneumonia, pleurisy, rheumatism, gastritis, measles, as the case might be.
>
> I had some of Fleming's *Tincture of Aconite* in my surgery and of this I put a few drops into a large bottle of water and gave it to the nurse of said children's ward with instructions to administer of it to all the cases of the one side of the ward as soon as they were brought in. Those on the other side were not to have the *Aconite* solution but were to be treated in the authorized orthodox way. . . . At my next visit I found nearly all the youngsters on the *Aconite* side feverless, and mostly at play in their beds. . . . Those on the non-*Aconite* side were worse, or about the same and had to be sent into hospital . . .
>
> And so it went on day after day: those that got *Aconite* were generally convalescent in twenty-four or forty-eight hours.
>
> . . . *Aconitum* in febricula was and is, my first reason for being a homeopath.[4]

Once fully persuaded by homeopathy, Burnett became one of its leading exponents at a time when, as he put it, "the social value of surgery is a baronetcy, the social value of homeopathy is slander and contempt."[5] With Dr. J. H. Clarke, Burnett studied with Dr. John Drysdale in Liverpool, where he built a successful practice during the years 1874–79. In 1879, Burnett moved to London, where he combined his own busy practice with working at the Royal London Homeopathic Hospital founded in 1850. With Dr. Robert Cooper and Dr. Thomas Skinner, Burnett and Clarke formed a London group to discuss therapeutics that became known as the Cooper Club. In addition, Burnett edited *Homeopathic World* and wrote some twenty-six books on therapeutics.

He took up enthusiastically Rademacher's organopathy, which Burnett called the "specificity of seat" of a remedy. An original and independent thinker, he was also an excellent clinician with a special interest in anatomy. Thus Burnett was well qualified to evaluate the worth of Rademacher's organopathy, which he defined as: "[t]he specific local action of drugs on particular parts or organs, as first systematized by Rademacher. . . . [I]t is a very convenient term in therapeutics as well as in aetiology and pathology."[6]

Burnett goes on to say that the term *organopathy* had been copied from Rademacher without acknowledgment, "but the real father of organopathy in essence and substance is . . . Paracelsus."[7] Burnett also saw its connection to homeopathy, like curing like: "[F]or a drug to cure the heart of its disease specifically it must necessarily affect the heart in some manner."[8] In fact, he describes organopathy as being of the nature of elementary homeopathy, but found that "some of the organ remedies of Rademacher posses a direct healing power over organ diseases that their provings in no way explain."[9]

Burnett asserts that the shortest path of curing occurs when the physician can successfully diagnose where the malady is located, because "the organ in the organism does indeed possess not only autonomy but hegemony, i.e., the organ is an independent state in itself, and in and on the organism exercises an important influence."[10]

Burnett also noted unexpected sympathies between organs: for instance, between the spleen and the male urethra; between the diseased eye (diplopia, ambylopia, and inflammations) and the poorly functioning liver; between the asthmatic lung and the spleen; between the retracted nipple and uterine or ovarian disease; and between the head and rectum.[11] Burnett recognized that homeopathic similarity could apply equally to the homeopathic similarity of the "totality of symptoms," as Hahnemann had emphasized, or to the affinity between certain organs and healing herbs. Burnett called all that he learned from Paracelsus and Rademacher "pure . . . therapeutically applied pharmo-dyanmics."[12] He developed the use of organ-specific remedies to a great degree and became "one of the most remarkable healers of modern times."[13]

Carl Friedrich Zimpel (1801–1891): Theosophy and Electrohomeopathy

Carl Friedrich Zimpel was a colorful and dynamic entrepreneur. He tried many occupational avenues before he found his medical vocation. Born in Prussia, he lived for many years in America, where he first made—and then lost—a fortune. He trained first as a railway engineer and then as a doctor, obtaining his medical degree in Jena in 1849. He began working and practicing in London the following year.

While in London, Zimpel encountered Swedenborgians and English theosophical circles, and these adherents introduced him to the works of Jacob Boehme, Jane Leade, and John Pordage and the millenarian doctrines of Joanna Southcott. Returning to Germany, Zimpel was inspired by the Swabian theosopher Johann Christoph Blumhardt (1805–1880) and the Romantic poet Clemens Brentano's short book on the visions of the stigmatic Anna Katharina Emmerich (1774–1824). Her visions of the Passion caused Zimpel to embark on a pilgrimage to Palestine.

Zimpel wrote more than twenty theosophical works with an expectation of a millennium, which he variously dated to 1866, 1873, and 1888. Back in central Europe, Zimpel continued his contacts with Blumhardt, forged a close friendship with Justinus Kerner, and met with the prominent *Naturphilosoph* and magnetist Karl von Eschenmayer (1758–1852) and the theosopher and professor of natural history Gotthilf Heinrich von Schubert (1780–1860). Thus Zimpel continued his study of therapeutics against a background of Pietistism, animal magnetism, and electrotherapy, which he had first studied in London. This was to form the basis of a quest that lasted the remainder of his life.

His homeopathic training began with Dr. Arthur Lutze, a homeopathic practitioner in Cöthen, Germany, but Zimpel first learned about spagyrics from a Frenchman, Henri Blanc, in Lyons in 1857. He was intrigued by the work of Christophe Beckensteiner, whose therapeutic method involved the delivery of remedies to the patient by means of an electric current. Zimpel's own textbook, *Die Reibungselektizität in Verbinding mit Imponderabilien als Heilmittel* [Electrostatics in connection with Imponderables as Remedies] (1859), asserted that this combination of electricity and homeopathy represented the zenith of the healing art.[14]

In Germany, Zimpel studied the work of Paracelsus and his followers, not only seeking out the best methods of working, but also trying to establish which herbs Paracelsus himself had used with most advantage. In the early 1870s, he began the manufacture and distribution of spagyric essences through German apothecaries in Leipzig and Göppingen. His work has been most influential, and is still the basis of some of the larger firms operating in Germany and Switzerland—those that continue to make spagyric essences while complying with the stringent government and EU regulations now in place.

In Zimpel's method, the phytotherapeutic herb selected is first fermented with water and yeast, a process that may last several days or weeks. Then, by means of a gentle steam distillation, the essential oils and alcohol are drawn off. The plant residues are then calcined to white ash, are mixed with distilled water, and are filtered. From this solution, the water-soluble salts are obtained. These electrolytes are then recombined with the essential oils and plant alcohol to form the spagyric essence.

Some purists object to fermentation on the basis that it adds something extraneous (yeast) to the phytotherapeutic herb. Nevertheless, it is the most practical way of obtaining the alcohol specific to the phytotherapeutic. Those who do not use this method usually have to use alcohol from wine as a supplement, because many plants do not produce enough alcohol without the fermentation process.

From 1868, Zimpel resided in Italy, where he became interested in the work of Count Cesare Mattei (1809–1896), the founder of electrohomeopathy, a combination of Hahnemann's theories and the notion of "vegetable electricity" based on spagyric preparations. By 1870, Zimpel had combined Mattei's ideas and his own to devise a range of remedies described in *Die vegetabilische Elektrizität zu Heilzwecken und die homöopathische-vegetabilischen Heilmittel des Grafen C.M.* [Plant Electricity in Healing and the Homoeopathic-Plant Remedies of Count C(esare) M(attei)] (1869). He continued to develop his spagyric ideas with reference to Paracelsus and, later, Johann Rudolf Glauber (1604–1668), alongside theosophers such as Friedrich Christoph Oetinger and Karl von Eckartshausen (1752–1803).[15] He organized the production and distribution of his remedies through German apothecaries, first in Leipzig in 1870 and then in Göppingen from 1873. Although Zimpel remained in Italy for the rest of his life, he corresponded almost daily with his agents in Germany to direct the manufacture of his spagyric remedies.

Zimpel's medical system could be regarded as the oldest spagyric system still in practice. It was inspired by Hermetic and theosophical ideas, although it was much modified along Paracelsian lines at the beginning of the twentieth century. His work influenced both the firm Phylak-Sachsen, currently operating in Switzerland, and Staufen-Pharma in Göppingen (Baden-Württemberg).

Cesare Mattei found his strongest succession in Germany, both through Zimpel and Theodor Krauss (1864–1924), a homeopath whose grandfather had been a pupil of Samuel Hahnemann. Krauss pioneered electrohomeopathy in Germany, and together with Johannes Sonntag (1863–1945), he founded ISO-Arzneimittel at Ettlingen

(Baden-Württemberg), today a major subsidiary of a large German pharmaceutical company.

Frater Albertus (1911–1984)

Albert Richard Riedel, also known as Frater Albertus and Albertus Spagyricus, was born in Dresden, Saxony, Germany, on May 5, 1911, and immigrated in 1929 to the United States, where he made his home in Salt Lake City, Utah. On his arrival in the United States, Riedel joined the Ancient and Mystical Order of the Rosae Crucis (AMORC), a neo-Rosicrucian organization for the dissemination of esoteric knowledge, founded in San Francisco in 1915 by the theosophist H. Spencer Lewis (1883–1939). Like the theosophical movement itself, AMORC held public lectures and courses on the esoteric tradition, and its influence on twentieth-century New Age movements has been considerable.

Following this model of public instruction (a notable aspect of the esoteric tradition in modern times as compared with secret societies in earlier periods), Riedel founded the Paracelsus Research Society in Salt Lake City in 1960 and the Paracelsus College-Utah Institute of Parachemistry in 1980. He carried on the alchemical tradition of his native country, infusing it with mystical Kabbalah and astrology, and he founded schools of alchemy in Australia and Europe. His stated goal was to improve the lot of humankind by giving access to hitherto secret teachings that had been passed on only through master and apprentice. The mission statement of the Paracelsus Research Society reads:

> It fosters the studies and researches of the arcane and physical sciences in the hope to contribute, by unbiased investigation and lawful demonstrations, to the knowledge extant. It teaches its findings to all free of charge or tuition. Its laboratory and classrooms are available to all regardless of race, creed, or nationality. Its purpose is strictly humanitarian. There is no membership.

Frater Albertus was the author of *The Alchemist's Handbook* (York Beach, Maine: Samuel Weiser, 1960), and his translation of the first German edition of *Praxis Spagyrica Philosophica* of 1711 was published by Samuel Weiser in 1998.

Manfred M. Junius (1929–2004)

Another contemporary German alchemist, the late Professor Manfred M. Junius, was born in Hagen, Westphalia, in 1929. After studying medicine in Germany, he traveled in Spain and the Middle East in search of living alchemical practice. He later settled in India, where he trained in Indian alchemy and Ayurvedic medicine. He became a professor of biology and also achieved distinction as a leading performer and judge of classical Indian *ragas* in the 1960s.

After returning to Europe, he worked with the Swiss alchemist Augusto Pincaldi (1918–1986) in Venice, and he made pioneering discoveries concerning nearly lost alchemical techniques of the late-seventeenth century. In particular, he pursued the Lesser Work, or Opus Minor, of the plant stone known as the *Circulatum minus,* following a recipe of Baron Urbigerus (1690). Andreas Libavius (1555–1616) defined the *Circulatum* as the "exaltation, of a liquor through a continuous dissolution and coagulation in the pelican with heat as the agent."[16] (The *pelican* was the vessel used for the process.) If the liquid plant stone is successfully made, it will separate a plant substance into its essential oil and the remaining body into its sulphur and salt without heat and almost instantaneously.

Manfred Junius was the author of *Spagyrics: The Alchemical Preparation of Medical Essences, Tinctures, and Elixirs,* and until his death, he ran his own practice and spagyric laboratory, Australerba Laboratories, in South Australia.[17] Junius gave regular master classes on alchemy in central Europe until his sudden death in 2004.

Contemporary Spagyric Pharmaceutical Companies

In Continental Europe, there are about a dozen major spagyric pharmaceutical companies whose methods of production are Paracelsian in character, although the methods of production of individual firms may differ slightly. These spagyric medicines, which are registered and recognized in the German Pharmacopoeia, are made in licensed laboratories in Germany and Switzerland to strict government and EU standards.

Demeter Georgiewitz-Weitzer (1873–1949), born in Baden, Austria, had been a leading editor and author in the German theosophical movement prior to 1914. In Leipzig, in 1907, he began publishing the influential monthly periodical *Zentralblatt für Okkultismus* (1907–1933) while simultaneously publishing his own works on modern Rosicrucians, Paracelsus, alchemy, and alternative medicine under the pseudonym G. W. Surya. He ran an extensive medical practice and continued writing about esoteric medicine throughout the 1920s and 1930s. He was interned by the Nazis for his interest in esotericism and opposition to the dictatorship. In the 1930s, Surya and Karl Richert (1896–1982), a spagyrist from Freiburg im Breisgau, founded Solaris-Labor (now called Solaria) in Baden-Württemberg. Work was interrupted by World War II, but Karl Richert continued production from 1954 until his death. Solaria is now under new management and has a subsidiary in Poland.

Alexander von Bernus (1880–1965), a poet born in Heidelberg, had extensive family connections with Goethe and the German Romantics and also founded the original Goethe Museum, now in Frankfurt. He was a close friend of Rudolf Steiner, who encouraged him in alchemical and medical research. His firm, Soluna, based in Donauwörth, in Bavaria, was continued after his death by his widow, Isa, and is now run by the Proeller family. The plants are grown organically in north Italy and are exported to Donauwörth for manufacture.

Conrad Johann Glückselig (1864–1934) was the inspiration for Phönix, in Bondorf (Baden-Württemberg). Trained as a chemist and natural scientist, Glückselig was also a theosophist and a student of Jacob Boehme. After 1914, he studied with Alexander von Bernus, and he developed his own spagyric medicine on the basis of Paracelsian principles. He subsequently founded Phönix Laboratorium, a major producer of spagyric and homeopathic medicines in Germany today.

Dr. (George) Gopalsamy Naidu is a research scientist involved in both conventional and natural medicines, and he is undertaking pioneering work in the treatment of cancer and other severe illness. He is a leading spagyrist who has conducted extensive research into the alchemical methods of Paracelsus and Carl Friedrich Zimpel, whose methods are applied in his spagyric pharmaceutical firm, Phylak Sachsen GmbH, based in Switzerland. George Naidu's work is supported by the EU, the German government, and a Swiss charity, Source of Life Foundation, which researches plants in their natural habitat and investigates their active healing properties.

Lemasor, a medium-sized pharmaceutical company located in Püttlingen (Saarland), was founded by Thomas Bönschen (b. 1953) in the late 1970s and now has subsidiaries in Venezuela and Pakistan. Following his university studies in philosophy at Marburg, Bönschen received instruction in alchemy and Hermeticism from two English alchemists in London who had long worked in a tradition deriving from G. R. S. Mead's Quest Society, an offshoot of English theosophy in the period 1909–1930. In the years immediately prior to their death in the 1970s, the Englishmen introduced Bönschen to a French Martinist group, and Lemasor is still close to French esoteric influences.

In 1974, Dr. Peter Beyersdorff founded Pekana, in Kisslegg, Germany, on the basis of homeopathic-spagyric remedies. The method of spagyric essence production involves adding yeasts and sugars to initiate fermentation so that the true plant mercury—the natural alcohol intrinsic to each particular plant—can be obtained. As described earlier, the tincture obtained is repeatedly filtered, and plant minerals extracted from the calcined plant are added. No steam distillation is used. The final step is potentization of the spagyric essence by hand succussion.[18] For Peter Beyersdorff, the role of the soul aspect in spagyrics is vital to the whole. According to him, "It was Paracelsus who said, 'Only a sick person becomes ill'":

Because of mental and emotional stress, the organs can become ill. This is completely logical, and I take this for granted in the development of diseases. Everything else is infection. But even infections are the result of a weakened immune system that has clearly been suppressed by an unhealthy mental or emotional state. The spirit is very important because the mind and body are one and cannot be separated. The cluster of bad information that is first felt by the soul affects the stomach, and this turns into information that harms the mucous membranes. Feelings and emotions are hurt, and this cluster of bad information is the first to enter the human body. This bad information causes chaos. Chaos is the opposite of order, and order and balance are necessary for good health.[19]

German complementary medicine research is still at the forefront of spagyric medicine, and there is increasing recognition in all branches of medicine that the mental and emotional aspects of a person's life play a major part in an individual's state of health. As Maximilian Bircher-Benner comments:

Disorder is illness. There is no illness that includes only the body but not the soul, even though this may not appear to be the case. The body and the soul are always ill together and both must be restored to health. Correct nutrition, detoxification and a healthy lifestyle, pure blood and good circulation, as well as fresh air and complete skin functions lead to an improvement of the organs and strengthening of the consciousness and thereby restoration of order and harmony. These are therefore the prerequisites for becoming healthy again in every illness.[20]

Spagyric medicine captures the full spectrum of healing potential in plants, including their remarkable empathy with human emotions. Through it, the soul and body can be healed.

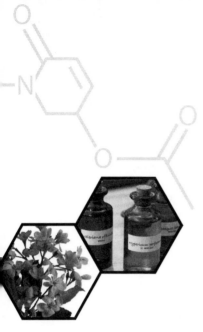

PART TWO

Praxis

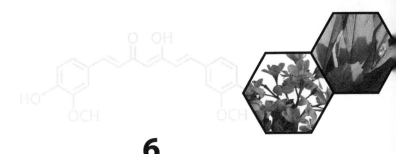

6

Making Spagyric
Essences

In describing the methods for making your own spagyric essences, I have tried to keep directions simple. There is already a great deal written about alchemy, and much of it leads away from the simplicity of the original intention: to maintain contact with the astral and vital healing powers of plants, to capture these powers, and even to enhance them.

A well-made spagyric essence is a liquid of delightful fineness. If we take time to make the essences well, we will be rewarded with tools of healing that will serve us well. Choosing an apposite time to make them according to the planetary disposition is ideal, but even more important is to make them while you are in a positive and cheerful frame of mind. Manfred Junius said it was important to make spagyric essences with love—just as it is important to cook with love for the family and friends who will sit around your table. Use meditation and prayerfulness to clear the mind, and free the heart of anxiety and resentment, for these will contaminate the essences. Let your shadow fall across them as little as possible, both literally and metaphorically. Far more can be achieved by working with conscious intention than by drifting along, thinking of other things.

Alchemical work is a point of departure rather than an arrival. The study of plants and the study of alchemy are both fascinating pursuits that are never finished. The Work is a continual process, both on the inner and the outer plane. Each of us must find our own way of working with herbs and drawing upon the great gifts that nature freely gives. The process of making even one spagyric essence brings with it a deepening awareness of ourselves and the world around us.

Even if you live in a city, you may still own enough outdoor space where you can grow some herbs in a container. Choose plants to which you are drawn, and pay attention to them—that is, do more for them than simply provide enough water. By observing their growth from seeds or cuttings, you can contact their healing forces. If you cannot grow your own herbs, make friends with plants whenever you are out in the countryside: take time to sit with them, and find out what you can about how they grow and how they respond to light and dark and the changing seasons.

As we have seen, spagyric essences differ from Flower Remedies and aromatherapy oils (sulphur) because they incorporate the salt (body of the plant) from which toxic matter has been purged. They also differ from normal herbal tinctures because they include the energetic information from the spirit or mercury of the plant in plant alcohols. We can select individual spagyric essences according to the rules of homeopathy and can combine them on the basis of general phytotherapeutic principles.

Ash in Spagyric Medicine

Carbonized vegetable material is itself a powerful restorative for low energy states, and the homeopathic *Materia Medica* includes a "corpse reviver" in the form of *Carbo vegetabilis,* or potentized charcoal. When a person exhibits a sluggish response, when he or she is chilly, lethargic, and weak, homeopathic preparations of *Carbo veg.* arouse the dynamism of the individual, working upon the whole economy of the organism, but especially on the digestive tract, the heart, and the venous circulation.

Charcoal is the residue of wood burned without air. The combustion process burns away methane and hydrogen, leaving mainly carbon (85–90 percent), with some volatile chemicals and an ash rich in potassium. Vegetable charcoal has been used for centuries to purify food and water, but activated charcoal absorbs toxic compounds from the body by means of its molecule-binding properties. Charcoal is not absorbed by the intestines, but as it passes through the digestive system, it can bind with toxins, waste products, and cholesterol toxins and help to move them out of the body. It has applications in the treatment of kidney patients who might otherwise suffer from high cholesterol and atherosclerosis. Activated charcoal in material doses and in homeopathic dilutions has been found to ameliorate flatulence and bloating.

Just as a flame may flare up and quickly subside, homeopathic *Carbo veg.* is also useful for those who experience a very sudden decline in energy and vitality. Though busy and energetic one day, the person's health may suddenly be broken the next, laid low by some virus or by shock. *Carbo veg.* is one of the most useful remedies for shock of any kind, including shock to the body caused by major surgery. In instances of shock, the body is very cold, the skin is clammy, and the face is pale. Despite this chilliness, a person in shock may wish to be fanned because of air hunger. There may be also be cyanosis with asthma. Due to shock, blood loss, or exhaustion following illness, there is stagnation in a patient's system, as though it was in the process of closing down.

As for the delivery of ash, some herbalists simply burn the plant they are using to make the tincture, and then add to the tincture a miniscule amount of ash—no more than sits upon the point of a knife. The spagyric process involves the calcination of the plant and then the recovery of the water-soluble salts by means of filtration and evaporation.

Making Your Own Spagyric Tincture without Distillation

This method is used when we work with fresh material such as freshly picked flowers or cleavers. (Skip the drying stage and cut up the plant material finely, using ceramic scissors.) It makes a satisfactory spagyric tincture when you do not have distillation equipment available, when you are working with fresh flowers that deteriorate rapidly after picking, or when the plant you are using has very little oil content.

Laboratory Equipment You Will Need

- A cutting tool; ceramic scissors are best
- A steel spoon
- A mortar and pestle
- A glass funnel
- Coffee filter papers to fit glass funnel
- Large, sterile glass jars in different sizes, and plastic lids—at least two or three jars that can be sealed and made completely airtight. If jars have metal screw-top lids, you will need plastic food wrap to prevent the corrosion of the metals from corrupting the spagyric essence.
- Sterile, dark glass bottles with airtight stoppers or screw caps
- Dropper bottles
- A 2-pint ceramic cooking pot, resistant to high temperatures
- A camping gas stove or a portable electric ring. The first stage of calcination will have to be completed outside, because it will create unpleasant smoke. Alternatively, you can build a fire outside using a framework of bricks or stones and firewood that will burn cleanly and well.
- Oven gloves
- A quarter of a pint (250 ml) high-proof alcohol (brandy or cognac). This is the *menstrum*. Buy the highest proof alcohol you can. Traditionally, red wine was distilled to make "spirit of wine," but nowadays this practice is illegal in many countries.
- Distilled water or fresh dew, collected and filtered.
- A notebook. It is always valuable to make detailed notes of your work as you progress. Your notes will be a tremendous resource to you as you persist. It is useful to keep accurate records of quantities, timing, temperatures, conditions of work, the time you started, the quality of the herbs, astrological aspect, weather, and so on.
- Labels. At every stage, always label the work with the date and time as well as the name of the plant.
- An astrological chart for the time of your work is a *sine qua non* for some. (This is, of course, optional.)

Harvesting Plants

If you have access to fresh, organic herbs, pick them at the optimum time: the plant should be at its best—healthy and mature. Select the day and hour of picking according to the planetary rulership of the plant (see chart on page 25). In additon, prepare yourself for the task: be sure you harvest mindfully and with gratitude for the healing energies of the plant. If you are working with the planetary rulership, begin work with a sun plant on a Sunday at the sun hour, and perform each stage at weekly intervals. This is not always practical or possible, of course, but timing is something to keep in mind.

Herbs should be harvested in dry weather, early in the morning—but not so early that there is still dew upon them. Leaves are usually gathered before the plant flowers are harvested. If you will be using flowers, then they should be picked when they open to full flower. Rhizomes should be gathered in the fall, when the leaves decline and the energy returns to the roots.

Old herbals were very particular about the timing of harvesting plants, and recent research has shown that the quality of plant constituents does indeed vary according to location and season and time of day, particularly with regard to the phases of the moon.

Phases of the Moon

New Moon

At the time of a new moon, the moon rises and sets with the sun; there is a balance of forces. Sap is high and there is an upsurge of energy. This waxing time is a good period in which to harvest Asteraceae, provided the flowers or herbs are ready. It is also a favorable time to begin a new project.

First Quarter Moon

At this time, energy is high and the sap is still rising. The moon rises at noon and sets at midnight. This is a good time to begin a new project, especially one aimed at alchemical transformation.

Full Moon

At this time, sap sinks in the stems of plants, but the electromagnetic energy is said to be at its height in living things. Two days before a full moon and at the full moon are good times for harvesting medicinal herbs—especially roots—while the sap is sinking.

Last Quarter Moon

This is the time to draw work to a close. Finish a project and begin to plan a new one. It is not a good time to harvest.

Drying Plants

Usually, you should work with dried herbs—with a few exceptions, such as cleavers, which should be used when freshly picked. Drying makes the amount of herb manageable to handle, and most of the material lost in drying is water, not precious oil.

To dry herbs, make sure they are clean and free of insects. Remove any blemished leaves, but leave whole leaves intact on the stem. It is important that the herbs dry thoroughly, with no traces of mold. Lay them out to dry in a single layer, ideally on a wooden frame with silk gauze or fine muslin stretched across it. Alternatively, you can tie them in small bundles and hang them where the air will circulate freely.

When dry, the herbs will have lost about four fifths of their green weight. Leaves should break cleanly and feel warm and crisp to the touch. If leaves are pliable, they are not dry enough; if they crumble into powder, they are too dry. Wash roots thoroughly before leaving them to dry, making sure they are not touching. Dry them until they break easily and cleanly.

Be wary of direct sunlight, because it will dry the herbs too quickly. Always store herbs away from full sunlight, which will fade their color and dissipate their vitality.

Ore et Labore

"Pray and work," the motto of St. Benedict (ca. 480–547), the founder of the Benedictine order, has become the motto of the alchemist, and the phrase is encapsulated in the word *laboratory*. The alchemist also purifies and transforms the self in the Work: for the true alchemist, the Work is never simply what takes place in the flask. There is always an acknowledgment that the attention and awareness of the practitioner plays a considerable part in making a successful spagyric essence that has captured the full spectrum of a plant's healing powers and its ardent, cosmic life force. A pure intention and a grateful heart are the alpha and omega of the Work. Prayers and invocations are traditionally said at the beginning of the Work. This one is an invocation attributed to Paracelsus:

> O Holy Spirit, show me what I do not know, and teach me what I cannot do, and give me what I do not have. Grant that you, O Holy Spirit, may dwell within my five senses; with the seven gifts you are to gift me, and I shall have your divine peace.
>
> O Holy Spirit! Teach me and show me so that I may live rightly with God and my neighbor.[1]

Mortar and Pestle

Most dried herbs must be broken up with a pestle in a mortar. To do this, work steadily and mindfully, methodically removing any stalks that are too tough to break down. When you have about a half pound (250 g), you can begin essence preparation. Keep extra dried herbs in brown paper bags stored in a dry place, or place them in large screw-top jars.

Maceration

Put the half pound (250 g) of dry, ground herb in a clean glass jar that is about 4 inches (10 cm) in diameter and about 8 to 10 inches (20–25 cm) tall. First, moisten the herb with a small amount of alcohol, brandy, or cognac. As the herb begins to absorb the liquid, you can pour on the remaining alcohol more freely to cover the herb and to leave ¼ inch (7 mm) of liquid above the plant. The jar should be no more than half full so that there is room for expansion and buildup of pressure. Seal the jar tightly, and store it in a warm place. Alchemists speak of the first degree of heat—just about the warmth required to hatch an egg, or just about body heat. Keep the jar in a warm room or on a windowsill, though some spagyrists prefer to keep the tincture in a dark place. To maintain darkness, you can put the jar in a box or wrap it in brown paper or foil.

Shake the jar daily at the appropriate hour, and leave it in its place for a minimum of two weeks. Some alchemists leave it for a lunar month or for forty days, the traditional period of waiting.

During this time, the alcohol will begin the work of separation, drawing out the sulphur (essential oils) and the mercury (naturally occurring plant alcohols). Circulation will begin as droplets condense on the sides of the jar and run back into the plant material. As the tincture matures, the color will darken. (The word *tincture* comes from the Latin *tingo,* "to color.")

Filtration

When the tincture is ready, first remove it from the warm place where you have been keeping it, and allow it to cool. Keep the jar closed. If you open the jar while the tincture is warm, some of the precious volatile oils will be lost. Filter the tincture into a dark glass bottle using a glass funnel lined with a coffee filter paper. When all the liquid has dripped through, seal the bottle well and store it in a cool place.

Calcination

Next, you can either take the herb-alcohol mush out of the filter paper and place it in a heat-proof casserole, topping it up with the dried herbs you have stored, or begin the calcination with a fresh batch of dry herbs. (I prefer the latter method, because it preserves the integrity of the plant.) Calcination should be performed out of doors; the smoke will be acrid and choking. Place the casserole on a hot fire or on a lit camping stove with the heat turned to high. Stir the herb mixture as it begins to smoke (keeping up-wind if you can). Eventually, the mixture will turn black—known as the *nigredo stage*. Continue to heat the herb mixture until it becomes pale gray or, preferably, white ash. (If you prefer, you can continue to the *albedo stage* indoors, because there will be no more acrid smoke.) Leave the ash to cool (and of course put out the fire safely).

Separation: the Preparation of Salts

Next, pour 2 pints (1 liter) of distilled water or collected dew over the ash and gently bring it to a boil. Then simmer the mixture gently for about 20 minutes, and after, allow the liquid to cool. Filter the liquid into a bottle. What remains in the filter paper is the death's head, the *caput mortuum,* which contains the heavy metals and toxic constituents of the plant. This should be thrown away or returned to the earth.

Calcination and Purification

Place the liquid into a clean, dry casserole dish and heat it again gently to just below the boiling point. As the liquid evaporates, the water-soluble salts remain. Leave them on a gentle heat for about an hour, then take them off the heat and allow them to cool. Add distilled water, and heat the mixture again gently, stirring to dissolve the salts. Cool, filter, evaporate, and calcinate for as long as it takes to make very pure white salt crystals. The greater the purity, the finer and more effective your spagyric essence will be.

Cohobation

Next, place the purified salts in a large jar and pour the tincture over them. You will notice a distinct change in the color and aroma of the mixture. Seal the jar tightly, and place it in a warm, dark place. Leave it for two weeks, then decant the solution into a dark glass bottle and seal it tightly. Label it clearly, then give thanks. This is the spagyric tincture. It is good medicine in its own right, but one final step will make it even better: In this next phase, which is called *exaltation, sublimation,* or simply *circulation,* the tincture is dynamized into a true essence.

Though a tincture will keep for perhaps several months, a well-made essence will keep for years.

Exaltation

The simplest method, if you have no distilling equipment, is to place the tincture in a large, sealed vessel so that the liquid takes up no more than half the space. This allows for expansion. The pelican, a vessel with two "arms," was the original alchemical equipment used for this purpose. If you live in a warm climate, you can simply place the vessel in the sun during the day and in the fridge overnight. In colder regions, place the vessel somewhere warm, such as an airing cupboard, during the day, and in the fridge overnight.

The point of this exercise is the rhythmic expansion and contraction of the fluid, which energizes the tincture in ways we do not fully understand. As it is warmed, the liquid volatizes and rises up into the space above, condenses again on the side of the flask, and then the droplets— sometimes called *sweat* or *tears* in alchemical texts—run back into the liquid. This rhythm can be continued for some time, allowing heating during the day and cooling and *relaxing* by night, and in this way, the essence concentrates its powers.

The process can be compared to the homeopathic remedy potentized by succussion, but with the tincture, there is no further dilution. Yet this rhythmic expansion and contraction seems to impart a higher vibration to the tincture. Practical experience demonstrates that the exalted essence is more energetic and has higher curative powers than the tincture, and it also has improved keeping qualities.

Exaltation can be performed as continuous evaporation by means of a reflux condenser: put the tincture in a flask and attach above it the reflux condenser. Heat the flask while allowing cooling water to flow through the condenser. To allow for still further expansion, an alembic can be mounted between the flask and the condenser. Keep the heat gentle so that this becomes a rhythmic process rather than a vigorous one. The circulation can be continued daily for a week or more. When the essence is ready, decant it into a dark glass bottle and seal it tightly. Label it clearly. Some people like to give their essences a special name.

Dose

A standard dose is seven drops in a little water, but you can adjust this according to need. If you have a very strong reaction to the essence, leave it alone for a day or two, then dose again with two or three drops. *Always* dilute a dose with water before taking it or administering it.

Paracelsus's Description of Making an Essence from Melissa

But the Primum Ens Melisae is prepared in the following manner. Take half a pound of pure carbonate of potash, and expose it to the air until it is dissolved (by attracting water from the atmosphere). Filter the fluid, and put as many fresh leaves of the plant *Melissa* into it as it will hold, so that the fluid will cover the leaves. Let it stand in a well-closed glass and in a moderately warm place for twenty-four hours. The fluid may then be removed from the leaves, and the latter thrown away. On top of this fluid absolute alcohol is poured, so that it will cover the former to the height of one or two inches, and it is left to remain for one or two days, or until the alcohol becomes of an intensely green color. This alcohol is then to be taken away and preserved, and fresh alcohol is put upon the alkaline fluid, and the operation is repeated until all the coloring matter is absorbed by the alcohol. This alcoholic fluid is now to be distilled, and the alcohol evaporated until it becomes of the thickness of a syrup, which is the Primum Ens Melissæ; but the alcohol that has been distilled away and the liquid potash may be used again. The liquid potash must be of great concentration and the alcohol of great strength, else they would become mixed, and the experiment would not succeed.[2]

Making a Spagyric Essence Using Distillation

Steam distillation is valuable for plants with a good amount of oil, such as *Rosemary* or *Melissa*. Some spagyrists consider steam distillation essential; others view it as too sudden and violent. These prefer the slow, steady maceration process.

Choices for steam distillation set-ups include a flask, condenser, and receiving vessel; or a Soxhlet extraction apparatus; or an oil separator with a flask.

Soxhlet Extraction

The advantage of this method of extraction is that it is a quick way to produce small amounts of tincture from plants where a water-only or alcohol-only extraction would be incomplete. Yet unless a vacuum pump is fitted, the extraction will be at a temperature that is higher than ideal, and some active principles may be lost.

Place finely ground herbs into the thimble (filter-paper cylinder), taking care not to overfill. Next, place the thimble in the Soxhlet chamber and assemble the equipment with a flask of water at the bottom and the reflux condenser at the top. The flask can be heated over a low flame or put into a sand bath or electric jacket. When the water has overflowed three or four times, a small quantity of alcohol can be added to the flask to extract those active qualities that are not water-soluble, and again, three or four passes can be completed.

Using an Oil Separator

This is perhaps the most elegant method of preparing an essence. Steam passes through the herb, releasing the volatile vapors, which are cooled in the condenser. As the volatile vapors become liquid again, they pass into the oil separator. The oil and water form two distinct layers, which can be drawn off separately. You can then move to the calcination of the plant using intact herb material.

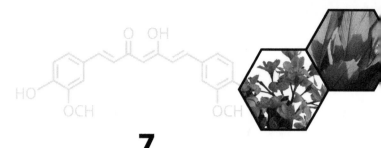

7

Plant Profiles and Therapeutics

Achillea millefolium

Asteraceae
Common name: Yarrow
Other names: *Thousand-leaf; nosebleed plant; milfoil.* The plant is known in French as *millefeuille;* in German, *Scharfgarbe;* in Italian, *achillea.*
Ruling planet: Venus
Parts used: Leaves, flowers

The Plant

Achillea millefolium is native to Europe but is widespread across all temperate zones. It is a perennial, aromatic herb growing in height to a couple of feet. The bipinate leaves, between two and four inches long, are slightly hairy and divided into fine leaflets, which grow in a graduated way, like a feather. They are broadest near the bottom of the stem. The white or pink-white flowers surmount an erect, furrowed stem that is up to two feet high and appears in late spring or early summer.

The plant is evergreen, so it is available for most of the year. It dries well if hung in small bunches where the air can circulate. It is a plant best harvested while flowering. Its fine leaves represent a large surface area, and the plant can accumulate toxins from the atmosphere, such as car exhaust, so choose your harvesting area carefully.

Sphere of Therapeutic Action

Nicholas Culpeper (1616–1654) attributes the knowledge of this plant to Achilles, after whom it is named and who had been instructed in its use by Chiron the Centaur. Achilles used it as a wound dressing for the fallen heroes of the Trojan War. It is a valuable styptic, quickly reducing bleeding from open wounds and stopping hemorrhages. Thought to have a special affinity for healing wounds made with iron, it has been called the soldier's woundwort, *herba militaris,* and knight's milfoil and has been used as a battlefield remedy for centuries. No special preparation is required; the leaves, stripped from the stem, can be packed in and around a fresh wound, and its antibacterial and antimicrobial action will set to work. It is also effective as a painkiller.

It has an extensive medicinal history among the North American Indians, who considered it a most sacred plant. The Blackfoot used it as an eyebath, the Winnebagos as an ear remedy, the Micmacs used it to sweat out a cold, and to the Navajo it was a medicine for toothache and ear ailments.

In the doctrine of signatures, its fine, feathery leaves resemble the blood vessels, branching out and becoming finer and finer, and indeed this is the sphere of its action. Taken internally, the spagyric essence helps to reduce hypertension by dilating the smaller blood vessels and the capillaries. It performs the same dilating function on the skin. During a fever, yarrow opens the pores and encourages sweating. Fresh leaves rolled up and stuffed into the nostrils will abort a nosebleed, and this use for the plant has led to one of its common folk names: nosebleed plant.

Achillea millefolium resolves congealed blood, so it can be used for clots, bruises, and bleeding beneath the skin or fingernails. It has even been known to be effective in aneurism and stroke. Its ability to relieve stagnancy in the blood means that it is also an excellent remedy for women: it regularizes the periodic flow, correcting it when the flow is too heavy or light and reducing clotting. Its normalizing effects may help to correct infertility in women, and it has the additional advantage of ameliorating period pain. As a styptic, it is useful in metrorrhagia and menorrhagia.

It is a soldier's remedy, a women's remedy: yarrow has been called a cure-all for its anti-inflammatory, antiseptic, astringent, carminative, tonic, and antispasmodic qualities. In Old English, it was called *gearwe,* meaning simply "healer."

The Salt Qualities of Achillea millefolium

Constituents: flavonoids, alkaloids, plant acids, and sesquiterpene lactones. The volatile oils contain azulene and glycoalkaloid achilleine. The plant contains salicylic acid, the original component of aspirin, and this may account for its use in fevers as well as its analgesic properties. Its ash content is less than 10 percent. Yarrow stimulates the lymphatic and vascular systems and is useful for removing toxins.

The Sulphur-Soul Qualities of Achillea millefolium

The essential oil has slightly spicy notes beneath a fresh, green, herby scent. Containing azulene, the essential oil collected by means of steam distillation is a wonderful blue color. The Chinese have also recognized its powerful spiritual qualities, which create balance between the yin and yang forces. Its sacred nature opens the recipient to intuitive perceptions. It brings about change through harmony, brings equilibrium to instability, and centers and stabilizes scattered energies. Its nature is to open the way to celestial flow, drawing in the energies of the sun, moon, and stars.

The warrior, no matter what his status in modern life, wants to be on the winning side. The warrior may experience resentment and anger from a wounding, whether this is the result of physical or metaphorical injury. He hates to be thought of as weak and finds it hard to deal with feelings of vulnerability. These reactions stimulate existential questioning: "Is life worth the struggle?" Yarrow, while gently nurturing and providing protection, may bring dreams and visions, putting the individual in touch with an intuitive understanding of their illness or situation in life.

Yarrow's ability to instill this visionary quality may be the reason why the long, straight, woody stems are traditionally held to be the most apt tools for casting the I Ching.

The Planetary Qualities of Achillea millefolium

"Being an herb of Dame Venus," as Culpeper quaintly puts it, the plant governs the reproductive cycle of women. Venus, the evening star and the only planet easily visible with the naked eye, is the light of this plant. It tunes the individual into balance. It also suggests that war is not always the best way to win what we want from life. Venus is love, and love can disarm the warrior.

Mars, the god of war, was the lover of Venus, goddess of love. In a beautiful painting by Sandro Botticelli called *Venus and Mars* (1485), a sleeping Mars is watched over by Venus, who is alert and composed. This throws light on how Venus might rule a knight's wound remedy. When the warrior is thrown back on his own resources, the light of Venus, goddess of love, is there to bring healing and peace.

Combinations

Achillea millefolium can be combined with most other herbs. It seems to intensify the medicinal action of other herbs.

Contraindications

It may irritate sensitive skin. Avoid use in pregnancy, because it can cause contractions. Avoid when breastfeeding and with small children under five years old. Large doses can cause vertigo or headaches in those who are susceptible.

Calendula officinalis

Asteraceae
Common name: Calendula
Other names: Pot marigold. In French, this plant is known as *souci*

des jardins; in German, *Ringelblume;* in Italian, *calendola;* in Spanish, *calendula.* The French marigold (*Tagetes patula*) is a different plant.

Ruling planet: Mars

Parts used: Leaves and flowers

The Plant

The plant is native to the Mediterranean countries, but it grows easily almost anywhere and has been naturalized around the world. It requires no special setting, and it readily seeds itself, though it prefers a bit of chalkiness in the soil or some loam. It is happiest in full sun. Its name, marigold or Mary gold, indicates its long association with the Virgin Mary—as for many healing plants—but its other common name is marsh marigold, from Old English *merso-meargealla.*

Like all the Compositae (the old name for the Asteraceae family), what appears as a single flower head is actually an inflorescence made up of tiny flowers, in this case, both disk florets and ray florets arranged in a sun shape. The color varies from deep yellow to rich orange. An annual plant, the common name *calendula* derives from Latin *calends,* the same root as for our word *calendar,* because of its long flowering period, from early spring through to the winter months. The leaves are long oblong or lanceolate and have small hairs on both sides.

The flowers can be eaten, and they look pretty added to salads. Boiling the flower heads produces a rich, golden-colored liquid, which can be used as a dye. In the past, this dye was used to enhance the color of butter and cheese and was used in cakes in place of more expensive saffron. A few florets dropped into a cup of boiling water make a refreshing, mild tisane.

Calendula was known in ancient India and later in ancient Greece as a therapeutic agent that was especially useful as a styptic and wound cleanser. It is the only herb that can be safely used to rinse a deep, open wound. It will speed up granulation and protect against bacteria. With calendula, however, wound healing can be so rapid that it is vital to make sure that the wound is properly cleaned. Foreign bodies such as grit can be trapped inside a wound and can cause problems later on. Not surprisingly, calendula has been a staple of battlefield surgeons through the centuries to prevent suppuration. Probably the last time it was used in quantity in this way was during World War I, when it proved its worth in the treatment of gunshot wounds.

Sphere of Therapeutic Action

This is perhaps one of the most useful of all therapeutic plants for its all-around medicinal qualities, its safety, and its wide availability. It is of inestimable value as a wound healer and belongs to the same family as arnica and *Bellis perennis,* but it is far safer than either, because, unlike arnica, it can be used even when the skin is broken. It is also antifungal, antibacterial, and antiviral. This is a wound remedy par excellence. Its spagyric essence should be given internally immediately following surgery or tooth extraction in order to stop the bleeding. It is styptic, antihemorrhagic, antiseptic, and anti-inflammatory.

Calendula spagyric essence can be taken internally for ulcers of the digestive tract and to build good-quality blood after excessive blood loss. It has antibacterial qualities against staphylococcus and streptococcus, so can be used as a mouthwash or gargle. Its styptic qualities make it useful for nosebleeds. It can be taken internally for lymphatic swellings or stagnancy in the lymph. A few drops of spagyric essence mixed into a mild aqueous cream is ideal for burns, including radiation burns, leg ulcers, and skin irritation as a result of varicose veins.

Calendula is safe for babies, and it is ideal for diaper rash and chaffing. New mothers can use diluted spagyric essence or cream on sore nipples, as well as on postpartum tearing or cuts. A few drops of spagyric essence added to a warm bath is soothing and healing.

The Salt Qualities of Calendula officinalis

In additions to its volatile oil, flavonoids, and triterpenes, calendula contains vitamin A, saponins, a yellow resin (calendulin), nitrogen, phosphoric acid, and silica. Its ash content is not more than 9 percent.

Silica, essential for healing skin and bone, is a valuable and necessary component of connective tissue and promotes epithelization. Silica builds strength of tissue, but it also helps to keep it elastic. Used after trauma, the silica in calendula ensures that scar tissue does not become too thick and tight, but remains smooth and elastic. Some studies have shown that silica deficiency is commonly found in coronary thrombosis patients. Internal use of calendula spagyric essence helps to maintain the elasticity of artery walls.

The Sulphur-Soul Qualities of Calendula officinalis

Calendulas like full sun and follow the sun in its daily voyage, turning their heads to gain maximum benefit. The flower heads close when the sun goes behind a cloud. On a psychological level, the individuals who are despondent when the weather is overcast or who suffer from Seasonal Affective Disorder (SAD) may find that regular use of the spagyric essence gives them a sunnier disposition. They may feel the cold rather intensely and are easily chilled. Anyone who feels markedly worse in damp, cold weather may benefit from a course of calendula spagyric essence to get them through the winter season.

The Planetary Qualities of Calendula officinalis

Calendula is ruled by Mars, the planet of war. Under a Mars aspect are soldiers, military surgeons, and physicians; people whose jobs may demand heroism, such as firefighters or police; and those whose jobs demand extreme physical endurance, competitiveness, and willpower, such as athletes and sports people. Mars relates to willpower, assertiveness, anger, ambition, and heroism. Mars energy is helpful for people who are frightened, filled with dread, anxious for the future, and fearful about some impending catastrophe. In anatomy, Mars rules the blood in all its aspects—the arteries and the blood cells; blood pressure and circulation; gall bladder and bile secretions; adrenal glands; muscles and tendons. Calendula is the premier remedy for wounds, amputations, and exhaustion after blood loss.

New research suggests that calendula may be useful as a treatment for HIV. Antitumor action in mice who have been given calendula essence has been reported, and in Germany, calendula is used in cancer cases.

Contraindications

Calendula can bring on contractions, thus internal use should be avoided in pregnancy. It is safe for external application, however, so can be used on stings, grazes, cuts, and burns in people of all ages.

Carduus marianus

Asteraceae
Common name: St. Mary's thistle
Other names: *Silybum marianum,* milk thistle. In French, this plant is called *chardon Marie;* in German, *Mariendistel;* in Italian, *cardo di Maria;* in Spanish, *cardo de Maria.*
Ruling planets: Jupiter (Culpeper) and Saturn
Parts used: Leaves and seeds

The Plant

These annual or biennial plants are native to the Mediterranean basin, Europe and East Africa and are naturalized in North America. They are edible, and, with the spiky parts trimmed off, the leaves impart to salads a refreshing, slightly bitter flavor. With their striking leaves, they have been cultivated as foliage plants as well as for medicinal qualities. St. Mary's thistle was described as the Virgin's milk because of the white veins on the leaves. Both St. Mary's thistle and Blessed thistle have been used as galactogues (that is, to increase the flow of milk), though Blessed thistle is now thought to be superior in this respect.

The name *silybum* is derived from the name *silybon,* given to thistle-like plants by the Greek physician Dioscorides. The deep green, spiny leaves of the milk thistle are glossy pinnates variegated with white veins.

The small purple flowers are followed by black seeds, each with a tuft of white hairs. As the seed matures, the plant diminishes.

The thistle has been cultivated for its leaves and also as a food. Thistles, however, also have a reputation for invading neglected spaces, ditches, and waste ground.

Sphere of Therapeutic Action

Known to Dioscorides, who considered it an antidote to snake bite, and also to Pliny, who recommended the juice mixed with honey as a liver cleanser, the thistle was also a popular remedy in the Renaissance. The eighteenth-century animist Georg Ernst Stahl (1660–1734) used the seeds to address respiratory complaints. Rademacher revived interest in the plant as a major organ remedy with a remarkable affinity for the liver and spleen, and it was also one of Count Mattei's favored medicaments.

Dull, aching pains in the hypochondria* are an indication for this remedy. Dull congestive headaches may also be an indication for this remedy, especially when accompanied by vomiting of bile. Rademacher noted that metrorrhagias, certain cases of sciatica, and some kinds of chronic coughs may all have their original seat of specificity in the liver or spleen. No remedy compares with this plant for addressing gallstone colic, according to Rademacher, but he concedes that this is difficult to diagnose. A useful tip from Rademacher: "[I]n all cases of abdominal pains . . . notice where the least remnant of pain lingers at the end of the attack; it is here that the primarily affected organ will generally be found."[1] In those who can benefit from milk thistle, the liver may be swollen more horizontally than vertically. (Vertical swelling indicates *Chelidonium majus*.)

Respiratory ailments associated with liver problems—such as asthma, a chronic dry, hacking cough that is worse at night, with stitching pains in the chest—can be helped by this remedy. Other symptoms

---

*In its anatomical sense hypochondria is the upper area of the abdomen lying below the ribs. It gave its name to imaginary disease, "hypochondria," because symptoms were often located in this area, often thought to be the seat of melancholy.

that may be aided by this plant: great fatigue and restless sleep that is broken by frequent waking, or by nightmares. Other indications: temperature regulation may be out of kilter, the person may be either very chilly or sweating upon waking, and he may sweat while eating at meal times.

The Salt Qualities of Carduus marianus

The plant has exceptionally high levels of cadmium. Silymarin has been found to increase superoxide dismutase (SOD) activity in both red and white blood cells, making it a more effective antioxidant than vitamin E. (SOD is an enzyme that repairs cells and reduces the damage caused by superoxide, the most common free radical in the body.)

The flavonolignans silybin and silymarin are antihepatoxic, and Gerard called it "the best remedy that grows for melancholy."[2] The active ingredient is highest in the seeds, as Stahl had realized. Silymarin, which is also found in lesser amounts in the leaves of this plant, is particularly concentrated in the seed coat. In Germany, the seeds are used as a specific antidote to mushroom poisoning, particularly by the aptly named death cap (Amanita phalloides), ingestion of which can indeed be fatal. Ash content is less than 10 percent.

The Sulphur-Soul Qualities of Carduus marianus

The individual may be easily angered or listless and absentminded. The person may walk into a room and forget what he came in for or forget what he was going to do next, or an individual may buy something in a shop and then leave it behind. However, thistles also have a reputation for invading neglected spaces, ditches, and waste ground. In chronic illness typical of disturbed liver function, such as in chronic alcoholism, the person will begin to neglect their surroundings as well as his or her person. Just as the plant keeps people at bay by its prickles, the sick may shun help for their condition, keeping their problems hidden, just as in the plant the seeds are hidden by white tufts.

The Planetary Qualities of Carduus marianus

The spleen comes under the dominion of Saturn and the liver under Jupiter, as Culpeper indicates. The expansive aspect of Jupiter must bend to the organizing power of Saturn, which strives to impose order and discipline in pursuit of structure and integrity. A person ruled by Jupiter has strong desires and can be an overdoer in every aspect of life. When the liver feels the strain of too much good living, the spleen tries to compensate in the short term before it too becomes exhausted. Saturn's positive quality is to preserve, to structure and order. It is responsible, enduring, and moral. It is often the case that when the liver is not functioning well, the spleen will also eventually suffer.

Contraindications

The plant is emetic in material doses.

Ceanothus americanus

Rhamnaceae
Common name: Ceanothus
Other names: Red root. In French, it is known as *céanothe;* in German, *Säckelblume;* in America, it is sometimes referred to as New Jersey tea, because the leaves were used as an infusion in the American War of Independence.
Ruling planet: Saturn
Parts used: Roots

The Plant

A shrub growing to four or five feet in height, this plant is native to North America but it has also been cultivated in Europe for the pretty, blue flowers of the cultivar. The North American genus has small, white flowers and is less ornamental. The ovate leaves grow to four inches long, and the stems are topped by panicles of tiny, cream-colored flowers. The root was used by the Cherokee Indians for the external treatment of skin cancer and venereal sores.

Sphere of Therapeutic Action

The appearance of the root of *Ceanothus americanus*—which has small nodules—suggests the lymphatic system, with its nodes. This plant was one of James Compton Burnett's principle remedies for the spleen. He wrote about it in his book, *Diseases of the Spleen* (1898), and it was widely taken up by both physicians and herbalists. Two years after Compton Burnett's book, a homeopathic proving indicated a definite affinity between this plant and the spleen. Traditional Chinese Medicine describes the energetic actions of the spleen, but it is an organ that has not been fully understood in Western medicine—and certainly not at the time Burnett was writing. In his *Erfahrungsheillehre,* Rademacher comments that spleen remedies are few and far between because spleen problems are not easy or straightforward to diagnose. The spleen is the largest organ within the lymphatic system, and although there may be pains in the spleen area (the left hypochondria), this is not the only guiding symptom that the spleen is underfunctioning. He noted a range of sympathetic symptoms from stomach pains to a cough, sometimes with asthma. There also may be dropsy, and there may be diarrhea or constipation as well. Rademacher also noticed that in women, spleen afflictions affected the uterus and gave rise to menstrual problems, or leucorrhea. Other presenting symptoms may include jaundice, with gallstone colic.

The spleen disorder manifests in edemas, heart weakness, shortness of breath, and physical and mental weakness. There is stagnancy. Ailments become chronic: chronic tonsillitis, grumbling appendicitis, lymph edema, dropsical swelling, and metabolic disorders. The spleen is an organ that separates waste products from reconstructive powers. It is necessary for the lymphatic system to function well to ensure the elimination of wastes that could compromise immune competence. In those with a spleen disorder, the spleen may swell enormously, and there may be deep-seated pains or a sense of fullness in the left hypochondria—so much so that the person will not want to lie on the left side. If the liver is also underfunctioning, the person may become anemic. In additon, there is great weakness so that the individual will not stand if he can sit and will not sit if he can lie down. There may be chilliness and shivering.

Whereas the use of the herbal tincture or low potency homeopathic tincture may cause aggravations, a course of treatment with the spagyric essence gently arouses the dynamism of the sick person.

The Salt Qualities of Ceanothus americanus

Plant ash of *Ceanothus americanus* has been found to be rich in potassium, calcium, magnesia, aluminium, iron, and silicon. This may explain the premature aging in people with spleen problems: deficiencies of these nutrients—particularly potassium, calcium, iron and magnesium—are frequently noted in the elderly. Depression is part of the deficiency syndrome associated with lack of calcium, iron, and magnesium. Decreased intercellular potassium has been noted in depressed patients who exhibit tearfulness, weakness, and fatigue. Constipation, edema, fatigue, and muscle weakness are all aspects of potassium deficiency.

The Sulphur-Soul Qualities of Ceanothus americanus

There is melancholy and purposelessness in the spleen patient. He may become rigid in his outlook and lose his sense of humor, growing melancholy and moralistic. In a negative state, responsibility—the negative pole of the idealism that shows in the healthy person—hangs heavily. They are overresponsible and fastidious; life wearies them with its perceived demands. On a psychological level, they experience stagnancy—lack of drive, lack of ambition. The individual may feel he has more to do in life, but he does not know what to be at. He goes on with the same job, unable to break free, but all the time he frets that his life is passing without his having achieved much. Ambitions that have seemed important in the past now seem to have served their turn. The individual wants something new, but does not know what. Everything that might appeal to him seems out of reach—too little money, too little time.

The Planetary Qualities of Ceanothus americanus

Saturn is Chronos, the god of time who rules entropy, limitation, aging, and decay. A negative Saturn condition is seen in the premature aging and running down of the energy of the patient. The hair may go gray or start falling out. The physical degeneration of someone with spleen and liver problems will be quite marked, with weakness, stiffness, and pessimism. Without correction, there can be a continual slide to chronic disease, cancer, rheumatism, and other such Saturnine diseases. Under a positive corrective remedy, the spleen regains its powers of separating wastes, which enables the body to regain control of its self-healing capacities—and the lymphatic system is key in this. The positive side of Saturn is the structuring and organizing principle that can reestablish order, correct elimination function, adjust mineral metabolism, and bring poise and optimism.

Chamomilla or Matricaria recutita

Asteraceae
Common name: Chamomile
Other names: In French, it is called *camomille;* in German, *Hundskamille;* in Italian, *camomilla;* in Spanish, *camomile.* It is often called German chamomile or "true chamomile," to distinguish it from Roman chamomile (*Anthemis nobilis*), which is a different genera altogether (and is called in French, *chamomille Romain;* in German, *Romisch Kamille;* in Italian, *camomila oderosa;* and in Spanish, *manzanilla,* meaning "little apple.")
Ruling planets: Mercury and Mars
Parts used: Flower heads

The Plant

Flowers should be picked in the morning or evening on hot dry days, when concentrations of the oils are at their highest. In wet weather, these can fall by 50 percent. Flowers must be dried carefully and thoroughly, because they are very susceptible to dampness in the air and may go moldy. Once thoroughly dry, they should be stored in airtight jars and used up quickly, because the valuable oil decays rapidly. If you purchase dried herbs, freeze-dried flowers (as compared to air-dried flowers) have been found to contain more oil.

Chamomilla is in the group of healing plants that includes *Achillea millefolium* and *Artemisia.* Originally native to Eurasia, it has naturalized in North America and Australia. While both chamomiles (German chamomile and Roman chamomile) have a therapeutic history extending as far back as the ancient Egyptians, Greeks, and Romans, German chamomile is stronger and has more medicinal uses, due perhaps to its larger amounts of volatile oils, which have a fresh, herby scent, a bit like mown grass. For aromatherapy and beauty purposes, Roman chamomile is often preferred for its fruity, sweet scent that is sometimes compared to apples. Both are calming. For centuries, Roman chamomile has been used to make fragrant lawns, because the scent rises as it is stepped on and the plant grows all the more vigorously for being trodden.

Aromatic *Matricaria recutita* is an annual with low-growing, hairy stems that branch into leaflets. From mid-summer to mid-autumn the white and yellow flowers appear. Each inflorescence rises on a single, erect stem that branches out from the main stem. Chamomile grows in dry soils and can break up hardened earth crusts. It is an excellent companion plant, sometimes known as "physician to the plants," because it has a strong influence on plants grown around it and the ability to revive flagging plants nearby. It will help transplanted plants to root successfully. It has a strong relationship to the earth, itself putting down deep roots.

Sphere of Therapeutic Action

The clue to its use lies in the word *matricaria,* which derives from Latin *mater* or *matrix,* meaning "womb." The plant is well suited to pregnant women and the ailments of small children, or for women during menstruation. Chamomile can be used to treat those who exhibit oversensitivity and irritability. A person—especially a woman—who could benefit from chamomile experiences pains that are intolerable wherever they are felt, and she may become frantic and may pace up and down. Such a person may fly off the handle, make unpleasant remarks, pick a quarrel, or be uncooperative, especially during pregnancy or menstruation. Stimulants, especially coffee, make this bad temper worse, as does being out in the wind and away from heat. Mental and emotional symptoms may come upon an afflicted person with great rapidity, and she may exhibit quarrels, sulks, and hasty words as she moves about hurriedly and with great impatience, not knowing which task to do first, picking up one thing and then moving on to the next, leaving the first task unfinished.

Dyspepsia, especially when it is the result of stress, is soothed by chamomile. Those suffering from dyspepsia may experience nausea and vomiting, resulting in anorexia to avoid the discomfort of eating. Chamomile is often required by both mother and child. An anxious mother will find her child does not nurse properly, and this in turn causes more distress. The chamomile child can be very demanding and wants to be carried. He may ask for some toy, only to throw it from him with great fury when it is presented. He demands food, only to tip it onto the floor. Because the mother is already tense and the child is inconsolable, the two will wind up each other. The teething chamomile child becomes frantic and cannot be pacified. His behavior may be quite frightening: stamping, kicking, banging his head, knowing no moderation. His typical appearance is that one cheek is red while the other is pale. He may be worse in hot, dry weather and better when it is mild or wet. Typically, the child is hot and very thirsty.

A few drops of essence added to bath water calms skin rash. You can work a few drops of the spagyric essence into an ointment or aqueous cream for applications to inflamed or irritated skin.

The Salt Qualities of Chamomilla

Chamomile contains relatively high levels of selenium, which is required for growth, resistance to infection, and good liver and pancreatic function. There are also high levels of calcium, magnesium, potassium, iron, manganese, and zinc. In addition to flavonoids and tannins, the volatile oil contains a number of highly specialized substances, including immunostimulating polysaccharides, which prime macrophages, and B-lymphocytes for wound healing. For those with many allergies, chamomile calms allergic reactions. Studies have shown that chamomile can markedly reduce gastric acid, which may help to calm the nervous system of the overcharged chamomile temperament.

Ointments containing the oil (alpha bisabolol) have been found to work better than hydrocortisone for skin inflammation.

The Sulphur-Soul Qualities of Chamomilla

The essential oil of chamomile contains azulene and is the most wonderful deep blue—the color of the Virgin Mary's cloak. Blue is calming, peaceful, and the color of spiritual aspiration. The essence assists in empathy and patience. After taking it, the person will be calm enough to talk quietly about a problem instead of railing at his or her fate. It encourages understanding and empathy with another person's point of view.

When used regularly, chamomile essence brings a mature outlook on life, so that what seems to be a life of hurried uncertainty assumes its true direction and purpose. It is helpful to meditate and practice mindfulness when taking the essence.

The Planetary Qualities of Chamomilla

In the negative state, a chamomile child demonstrates the restlessness and changeability of Mercury with the irritability of Mars. Without adequate powers of reasoning and expression, the child is temperamental and overreactive. Even in sleep, there may be signs of distress or the individual may weep without waking, which shows that the disorder goes deeply into unconscious processes.

Mercury is the messenger of the gods. Acting as a go-between for earth and heaven, he promotes communication between the terrestrial and celestial realms. Blue—the color of the essential oil of chamomile—is the color of the throat chakra, which governs communication, expressiveness, and spiritual growth. The small child learning to speak, understand, and express himself, is under the influence of Mercury. Where there is confusion, the powers of logical reason, empathy, negotiation, and self-expression in constructive dialogue are the gifts of this planet. This shows in chamomile's ability to cooperate and support other plants around it. The Mars aspect promotes healthy assertiveness in place of unreasoning aggression.

Crataegus oxyacanthoides

Rosaceae
Common name: Hawthorn
Other names: White thorn. The plant is called in French, *aubépine;* in German, *Hagedorn;* in Italian, *marruca bianca;* in Spanish, *espina blanca.*
Ruling planets: Sun and Mars
Parts used: Flowers, leaves, and berries

The Plant

In Greek, *kratos* means "hard," *oxus* means "sharp," and *akantha* means "thorn." *Haw* is an old English name for "hedge," and *Hagedorn,* the German name for *Crataegus oxyacanthoides,* means "hedgethorn," so this plant has a long association with boundaries. The Greek name is accurate: the wood is hard and the thorns are long and sharp; it is not a hedge you can brush past. Hawthorn was planted to ward off sickness and evil. It is also known as May blossom for the time of its flowering. The white flowers give a very bridal air to the countryside when the hedges are in flower and a very distinct scent fills the air. Hawthorn is a vigorous plant that can live to a great age. When the wood is burned, its temperature is the hottest of any wood.

The deciduous plant forms a shrub or small tree, with spreading branches and sharp thorns that are three quarters of an inch long. The leaves are deeply lobed, glabrous, and broad-ovate or obvate and are up to two inches long. The scented white flowers, which appear in May, are arranged in clusters of about a dozen. (A cultivar, similar in all respects to the species, has flowers of a very deep pink.) Flowers are followed by the egg-shaped scarlet fruit of the hawthorn berry. The plant is found widely across the northern temperate zones of Europe and has become naturalized in North America.

Sphere of Therapeutic Action

One of the oldest known medicinal plants, hawthorn has a long therapeutic history and was already known by Dioscorides as a heart tonic. In recent years, the plant has established a record of confirmed safety, with clinical evidence to support its cardiotonic activity. These studies are based upon mixtures of leaf and flower or leaf, flower, and berry. There may be a synergy between the flowers and leaves or among flower, leaf, and berry that has yet to be explored. There have been no clinical studies on the benefits of the berries alone.

This is the preeminent heart tonic, safer than digitalis (which is actually a heart poison and may have cumulative toxic effects; hawthorn is ideal when digitalis-based products are not tolerated). For some of those who may benefit from hawthorn, the pulse is rapid and weak, and there may be dyspnea (shortness of breath) and dropsy. Hawthorn strengthens the heart muscle, and as a result blood pressure may be decreased. In the person who needs hawthorn, there may be symptoms of high blood pressure and angina pectoris, with pains in the left chest and under the left clavicle.

Hawthorn is useful not only for heart disease itself, but also for the fear of heart disease, which may discourage an individual from taking enough exercise to strengthen the heart. He may feel that heart failure will follow any exertion. Because excitement brings on a range of symptoms, from cold hands and toes to headache and weakness, the thought of exertion may bring on a hypertensive state almost as much as actual activity. For such a person, there may be a hurried feeling due to the rapid action of the heart, which is typical in those who may be angry, irritable, and cross. Hawthorn acts as a sedative and brings calm.

The Salt Qualities of Crataegus oxyacanthoides

The fruit contains saponins; glycosides, including flavonoids; ascorbic acid; and other acids.

The essence is said to have a dissolvent effect upon calcareous deposits in the arteries. Culpeper lists it as a remedy for dissolving stones and gravel of the kidneys and the bladder.

The ash contains calcium, phosphorus, potassium, and magnesium. Potassium is often found in plants that are diuretic, and recent research shows some correlation between lack of magnesium and heart arrhythmias.

The Sulphur-Soul Qualities of Crataegus oxyacanthoides

The thorn associated with Joseph of Arimathea that flowers at Glastonbury, in England, is a specimen of hawthorn. By tradition, the hawthorn is a holy plant associated with suffering: legend makes it the source of Christ's crown of thorns. The heart of the hawthorn person may be broken from grief, sorrow, or long-sufferings. Despair and fragility are keynotes. The individual may develop strategies for keeping people at arm's length, just as the plant itself maintains boundaries with its sharp thorns.

The person with chronic heart afflictions tends to close down from a painful world and desires to keep completely quiet, yet even this shows a resistance between the self and a threatening world. This resistance sets up a tension between the flow of blood and the walls of the vessels that contain it. When the walls of the blood vessels are too constricting, the result is hypertension. Hawthorn strengthens the heart muscle, clears the arteries, and makes the blood vessels more elastic in order to withstand heart irregularity.

The Planetary Qualities of Crataegus oxyacanthoides

The sun warms, relaxes, releases, and stimulates growth. It powerfully affirms all life, and, as the most generous being in our solar system, it unceasingly spends itself for the benefit of living things. In alchemical imagery, the heart is the sun of the body. The heart must be warm in order to relax and to release tension. It can stimulate spiritual growth by opening to love and compassion—for the suffering self as well as for others. When we describe someone as open or warmhearted, we contrast this with the closed, coldhearted person. These warmhearted people are approachable, life-affirming, loving, and giving. They too may have suffered grief and sorrow, but their "sun" remains open and giving. Just as the hawthorn has a thorny side, Mars, associated with aggressive behavior and suppressed anger, can be an important factor in heart arrhythmias. Nevertheless, in the Greek myth, Mars is disarmed by love.

Equisetum arvense

Equisetaceae
Common name: Horsetail
Other names: The plant is known in French as *equisette;* in German, *Ackerschachtelhalm;* in Italian, *rasperella;* in Spanish, *belcho.*
Ruling planets: Venus and Saturn
Parts used: Leaves

The Plant

Widespread in North America and Eurasia, this plant is thought to be extremely ancient and one of the main trees of the Carboniferous age (270–370 million years ago). Fossilized traces of this once huge tree (60 feet tall) can be found in coal. It has hardly evolved: once a tree but now a rush, the present-day plant, though much smaller, is otherwise almost identical to its forebear. Its habit is fernlike; it spreads by spores and has no leaves or flowers as such. In spring, deep underground rhizomes push up the tall stems, which are soft and bare. When these die back, they are replaced by erect, hollow, segmented stems—a bit like bamboo—with long, narrow leaves that shoot from the nodes. The soft spore stems can be eaten and were used by the Romans—but for medicinal purposes, it is better to wait for the silica-rich hard stems of summer.

To use the leaves, pick them in early summer and dry them quickly to keep them green. Discard them if they turn brown. Crushing them with a rolling pin to break down the fibers helps moisture to escape the leaves and speeds the drying process.

Sphere of Therapeutic Action

As a beautifier, this silica-rich plant strengthens the nails and hair and is ideal for those with brittle nails or split ends. It promotes smooth, elastic connective tissue and helps to repair tissue both inside and outside of the body. As such, it is excellent for postoperative use or after injury. It assists in the absorption of calcium and helps to keep the bones and the skeleton strong, thereby aiding the strengthening of weakened joints. It is good for postmenopausal women with thinning bones, and it is also useful for repetitive strain injury. As a wound healer, it slows bleeding, cleans pus, and clears infection. Mildly diuretic, horsetail's reputation is as a cleanser that strengthens the arteries and veins and removes buildup of deposits of uric acids and cellulites. In this way, it has earned the nicknames of nature's Hoover and "bottle brush."

In the horsetail individual, there may be a constant dull pain and a constant desire to urinate, which does not relieve the pain. It is almost specific for cystitis in adults, and it is an excellent remedy for children who suffer nocturnal bedwetting from nightmares. For those who may benefit from horsetail, pains are dull and heavy and are worse on the right side of the body and affect the lower back. Some of these may be rheumatic pains that run down the outside of the leg almost to the knee.

The Salt Qualities of Equisetum arvense

The raw plant contains 30 percent silica, while the ash contains a phenomenal 70 to 80 percent silica, soluble in water and in alcohol. Other constituents include flavonoids, alkaloids, phytosterols, saponins, nicoyine, palustrine and palustrinine, silicic acid, selenium, and zinc.

The Sulphur-Soul Qualities of Equisetum arvense

Equisetum clears blockages on all levels, strengthens the will, and gives structure and organization to life. Pain in the limbs, the lower part of the body, and persistent headaches are a continual reminder of the frailty of the material body. The frequent need to urinate can limit the activities of horsetail individuals. Continually battling with fatigue, they feel better after an afternoon rest. These people may be irritable or fearful of life and what it asks of the individual. Just as the plant itself is not highly evolved, the horsetail individual has trouble evolving, or moving on. Horsetail will assist the in transmuting the inner qualities of self into the higher spiritual virtues.

The Planetary Qualities of Equisetum arvense

Saturn rules the bones, teeth, and joints. In addition, the spinal column, with its ligaments and its alignment, comes under this planet's governance. Saturn also relates to Chronos, the god of time, so many of horsetail's therapeutic effects are for those of late middle age. The Saturn aging cycle begins in the late fifties, a time when bones weaken and joints stiffen; when uric acid may build up in the extremities, causing gout; and kidney energy begins to fail.

Saturn brings in responsibility, order, integrity, and endurance. Beginning in the late fifties, the Saturnian phase of life is a time of consolidation of patterns that were established in youth—but these can go too far. Rigidity, fixed ideas, and closed thinking can begin to dominate. Life's opportunities may begin to contract. With bones and joint mobility weakened, this time of life can be the beginning of restriction and limitation. Steps must be taken to remain flexible, outgoing, and ready for new adventures in life. It is important for such an individual to remain connected to the present, to keep active and interested in his own affairs, and not to accept decline and limitation.

Contraindications

Because of its heavy mineral load, prolonged use of horsetail can burden the kidneys. It can be used in staggered treatments—one week on, one week off—for some months, or taken for a month with an interval of several days before another course of treatment.

Foeniculum vulgare

Apiaceae (formerly Umbelliferae)
Common name: Fennel
Other names: In French this plant is known as *fenouil;* in German, *Fenchel;* in Italian, *Finocchio;* in Spanish, *hinojo*
Ruling planets: Mercury in Virgo (Culpeper)
Parts used: fresh or dried leaves; seeds

The Plant

From its native habitat by the Mediterranean, this plant has spread across Europe and Asia and is now widely naturalized elsewhere. It was cultivated as a vegetable in classical antiquity for the edible white bulb with its delicate flavor of aniseed. Charlemagne (742–814) encouraged agriculture throughout his great empire and caused fennel to be cultivated on all the imperial farms from the River Elbe in the north to the Ebro in Spain. In this way, the plant became naturalized throughout northern and central Europe. Although the fennel plant has a preference for dry, sunny coasts, it will grow anywhere, even on rough wasteland. It is a tall perennial or biennial plant, and the erect, hollow stems with pinnate foliage divided into fine leaflets look extremely decorative in gardens and flower arrangements. The umbels of tiny yellow flowers bloom in summer, followed by gray-brown seeds. Fennel closely resembles the dill plant and will cross-pollinate with it if the two are planted too close together.

Sphere of Therapeutic Action

The fennel seed is stomachic and carminative, useful for indigestion and flatulence. As an aromatic herb, it was known to the ancient world as a digestive. It gently stimulates the liver and encourages bile production for improved digestion, especially of fats and fried foods. Its action is effective, yet gentle enough for babies to tolerate; therefore fennel is a favored ingredient in many gripe waters.

The ancient Greeks knew the herb as a remedy for corpulence and today it is still thought of as a slimming aid; it reduces bloating and the sensation of fullness or heaviness in the stomach after eating, especially after rich food.

It is a warming herb and this heating quality helps digestion, improves mood, and tones the whole system. The Romans gave fennel to athletes, believing it strengthened and toned the muscles, as well as giving courage. Gerard recommends fasting on fennel tea in order to strengthen the eyes, and Hildegard of Bingen thought fennel especially suitable for eye troubles in people with blue eyes. The spagyric essence can be taken internally as well as used as an eyewash or compress for conjunctivitis or just to refresh eyes tired by too much work at the computer screen. Its regulating properties will also assist in beautifying the complexion and it is especially useful for skin that is too oily. Fennel is a galactagogue, helping to regulate the flow of milk in nursing mothers.

The Salt-Body Qualities of Foeniculum vulgare

For thousands of years fennel has been recognized as a digestive, and recent research has shown that the anethole and terpenoids found in fennel inhibit spasm in the smooth muscle of which the digestive tract is composed. This is thought to account for fennel's carminative properties. Its ability to regulate the digestive secretions makes it useful for the control of hyperacidity. The anetholes in fennel have been shown to have antimicrobial properties, and the spagyric essence may be helpful in cases of *Salmonella enterica* and candida, thrush, and other conditions of yeast or fungal origin.

As it has a diuretic action and contains appreciable amounts of potassium, the spagyric essence may be helpful as an adjunct therapy in hypertension. Frenchone and anethole have been found to have expectorant properties, making fennel a useful herb for the relief of catarrh; and it is also safe for use by small children with respiratory congestion. Other constituents are limonene, a natural botanical insecticide and oil solvent; phelandrene, anisic acid, camphene, a-pinene, tannins, sodium, magnesium, and calcium.

The Sulphur-Soul Qualities of Foeniculum vulgare

Fennel was one of the favorite herbs of Hildegard of Bingen who considered it an excellent antidepressant. In addition to its carminative properties, settling the digestion, it also sweetens the breath and acts as a natural deodorant. Hildegard suggested fennel preparations as a massage for the relief of melancholy recommending its application to the temples, nape of the neck and the entire body, especially the solar plexus, to alleviate depression.[3]

It reduces stress, and produces a lightening of mood. Fennel works on the physical and mental-emotional aspects of the human being, bringing strength and quiet joy. For those who are finding everyday life more exacting and fatiguing than it need be, fennel enhances energy and confidence and provides protection from unwelcome outside influences. Fennel provides courage and endurance in adversity.

The Planetary Qualities of Foeniculum vulgare

Fennel is widely used in cooking to make fish more digestible for, as Culpeper claims, "it consumes that Flegmatick humour which Fish most plentifully afford and annoy the body by, therefore it is a most fit Herb for that purpose though few that use it know why or wherefore they do it, I suppose the Reason of its benefit this way is because it is an Herb of Mercury and under Virgo, and therefore bears Antipathy to Pisces."[4]

Contraindications

Generally fennel is thought to be very safe but extremely large quantities may disturb the nervous system, and it should be avoided in epilepsy. Fennel is a galactagogue, so pregnant women should avoid it in case it brings on milk production too early.

Combinations

A combination of rosemary and fennel is enlivening, bringing mental clarity and improving concentration and memory.

Galium aparine

Galiaceae or Rubiaceae
Common name: Cleavers
Other names: Goose grass, bedstraw. In French, the plant is known as *gratterton,* in German, *Klebelabktaut;* in Italian, *cappelo da tignosi;* in Spanish, *presera.*
Ruling planets: Venus and Saturn
Parts used: Fresh shoots

The Plant

Native to North America and Eurasia, the plant has naturalized in the southern hemisphere. Classified by Linnaeus, Rubiaceae consists of some three thousand species, including the bedstraws, but also including important food plants such as *Coffea arabica.* Dried and roasted, the seed heads of *Galium aparine* can also be used as an ersatz coffee.

Two leaves grow together with four *stipules,* two to each leaf, which mimic the leaves, and this cluster forms rosettes or whorls on slender, angular stems. The flowers are small, four-petalled stars. After the flowers come the seed heads, small globes with hooked bristles that can rapidly attach themselves to any passing human or animal. (*Aparine* is from Greek word meaning "to seize.") In this way, the plant spreads itself widely over a region: angular hooks on the stems attach themselves to anything that passes—the inspiration for Velcro. By means of these hooks, the plant can force its way through dense vegetation. The plant stems will also stick to themselves, and in the past the plant was used to make impromptu baskets and sieves for milk. Look for it from February onward, showing itself as a dense mass of bright green leaves. In its rampant growth we can see its vitality. In summer, small, white, four-petaled flowers appear and then the plant will begin to stick. If you can find very young, new shoots, you may chop them finely and add them to salads for a tonic. Later, as the plant matures, the stems become tough and hairy, and once the seeds arrive, it is no longer useful medicinally.

Sphere of Therapeutic Action

Pliny and Galen recommend cleavers for keeping slim, and Gerard claims it is a marvelous remedy for snakebites and insect stings. From at least the thirteenth century, it has been known as a blood cleanser and tonic, and from at least the fourteenth century, it has been used to make ointments for skin inflammations, burns, and scalds. In the ancient world, it was thought to be a cancer remedy.

Cleavers is a prime example of a common weed despised by gardeners that has gentle but highly effective cleansing and toning powers. It makes an excellent spring tonic. Animals know this: hens, horses, and sheep will happily consume it. It acts on the urinary system: it is a diuretic for dropsy, and it removes gravel and stones from the urinary tract.

Said to have the "power of suspending or modifying cancerous action, it has a clinical record for use for cancerous ulcers and nodulated tumors of tongue."[5] It promotes cellular renewal of the skin and promotes healthy granulations of ulcers.

By promoting lymphatic flow, *Galium aparine* assists in the removal of metabolic wastes, and it is excellent for swollen glands, adenoids, tonsillitis, and glandular fever. It is safe for young children with swollen glands around the neck and throat. Its reputation for helping to shrink tumors is due to its powerful cleansing effect: it cleans and soothes the urinary system and relieves the burning pains of cystitis, chronic urethritis, kidney inflammation, irritable bladder, and prostate problems. If taken as a lymph cleanser in the spring, cleavers makes the skin appear radiant and well nourished. The essence can be used as a mouthwash and gargle for sore throats and tongue problems.

Medicinally, *Galium aparine* works best when fresh; it is not as effective used in dried form. Freshness makes it ideal for an annual spring detox after the winter months. It can be picked in spring and used daily: It can be juiced and added to smoothies and fruit or vegetable drinks—or, if a juicer isn't available, its small shoots can be chopped finely, put in a polythene bag, and crushed with a rolling pin so that the juice can be wrung out of the plant. The leftover mush can be used on skin inflammation, burns, sores, and blisters or can be used as a cooling aid whenever the skin is hot and red. It is also cooling and soothing for psoriasis sufferers.

The Salt Qualities of Galium aparine

The plant contains anthraquinone derivatives, flavonoids, iridoids, and polyphonic acids. Asperuloside, a substance that the body converts into prostaglandins—hormonelike compounds—affects the blood vessels and may stimulate the uterus.

The Sulphur-Soul Qualities of Galium aparine

The negative aspects of cleavers arise from congested thoughts and irritability, especially over minor things. The person may be quite spiky, capricious, and fidgety. He may fret about the small things and may have an edgy, nervous, high-strung disposition. Urinary frequency often accompanies this nervous disposition. Cleavers helps to clear the moody, fearful, weepy, or self-pitying tendencies, bringing instead a contented, lighthearted approach to life.

The Planetary Qualities of Galium aparine

Venus rules the water economy of the body: the genitourinary system, the hormonal system, the gonads, the veins, and the tongue. All kinds of kidney problems and dropsy come into her province. Cleavers removes the Saturn tendency to stagnation in the lymphatic system, cleansing and relieving the congestive and rigidifying tendencies of Saturn. It is beneficial to the bones, ruled by Saturn, as well as to the arteries, sinews, lymph, and nerves. In fact, wherever there are long, tubular structures in the body—all ruled by Saturn—cleavers will clear them, flushing the toxins out through the urinary system. Saturn governs eliminative functions, the bones, joints, ligaments, the spinal column, neck, limbs, and the skin. Cleavers streamlines the body, lessening edemas and restoring the clean lines of the facial contours where there was swelling, especially around the eyes. As a result of taking cleavers, the neck may be smooth, without the lumpy nodules of congested lymph glands.

Combinations

Galium aparine can be combined with *Taraxacum* (dandelions—roots and leaves) and *Urtica dioica* (nettles).

Contraindications

Galium aparine is generally safe and nontoxic. Because it is a powerful diuretic, however, caution should be exercised with regard to diabetics and those on heart medications.

Hypericum perforatum

Clusiaceae
St. John's wort
Other names: In French, it is called *mille pertuis;* in German, *Tupfelharten;* in Italian, *perforata;* and in Spanish, *hierba de San Juan.*
Ruling planet: Sun
Parts used: Whole plant

The Plant

Hypericum perforatum is an herbaceous perennial native to Europe and naturalized in North America. The pale green leaves are sessile, branching out directly from erect stems. Pellucid oil glands run along the edges of the leaves and appear as perforated dots when held up to the light, which give rise to the name *perforatum*. With five sepals and five petals, the flowers are bright yellow, and the plant flowers throughout the summer. Traditionally, however, the time to pick the flower is on St. John's Day, June 24, just after the summer solstice (June 21).

Hypericum is Greek for "over apparition." It was thought that the plant would cause evil spirits to fly away, which ties in with its reputation as a nerve tranquilizer and antidepressant. In some sort of corroboration, Paracelsus comments on *Hypericum perforatum:*

> The veins upon its leaves are a signatum, and being perforated they signify that this plant drives away all phantasmata existing in the sphere of man. The phantasmata produce spectra, in consequence of which a man may see and hear ghosts and spooks, and from these are induced diseases by which men are induced to kill themselves, or to fall into epilepsy, madness, insanity. . . . [T]he Hypericum is almost a universal medicine.[6]

Sphere of Therapeutic Action

The essential oil is red and the tincture is blood red: signatures that *Hypericum perforatum* is a venerable wound remedy, especially for those areas rich in nerves. Thus it is useful for fingers crushed in car doors, falls on the coccyx, and tooth extraction. Analgesic, anti-inflammatory, and antiseptic, *Hypericum perforatum* is used for burns, sores, wounds, cuts, bruises, and bites and stings. There is anecdotal evidence that prompt use of *Hypericum perforatum* can prevent tetanus. A leading symptom is shooting pains in any part of the body, especially following an injury. If there is an injury to a finger and the person has shooting pains up the arm, *Hypericum perforatum* may be indicated. Pins and needles, as well as chronic pain, are also symptoms that respond well to this remedy.

A special sphere of action is the nervous system: depression; hypersensitivity; chronic illness; neuralgias; violent pains (from any nervous cause); nervous exhaustion; and melancholy, especially in inclement weather, are all indications for a course of St. John's wort. Fears and anxiety may manifest in bladder problems, headaches, insomnia, hypersensitivity, and stress. It will have a resolvent and expectorant effect on chronic pulmonary problems.

The Salt Qualities of Hypericum perforatum

Among several minerals, *Hypericum perforatum* contains the planetary metals iron, mercury, copper, and lead. Constituents are: red hypericin, astringents, and flavonoids. Hyperforin, a key constituent, has been found to be protective against gram-negative bacteria and is being researched for reducing alcohol addiction. Hyperforin is thought to inhibit serotonin reuptake, so it may work on depression in a similar way to selective serotonin reuptake inhibitors (SSRIs). Several trials analyzed by the Cochrane Institute have demonstrated that *Hypericum perforatum* is more effective than placebo and more effective than many drugs in the treatment of depression. These studies tend to work on the assumption that there is a single active ingredient that can be isolated, rather than a synergy from within the plant, so the effects they measure may be much weaker than those of spagyric essences, which capture the healing potential of the entire plant.

The Sulphur-Soul Qualities of Hypericum perforatum

The person may be imaginative and creative, but for various reasons, he does not express that creativity, and this repressing of an essential part of the personality may lead to the depression with which this plant is associated. These feelings may be exacerbated in the winter months, when the shorter days seem to impose further limitations. The vitalizing principles of *Hypericum perforatum* bring qualities of energy, will, self-expression, and dynamism of the personality. St. John's wort shines a new light on old problems, promotes positive thinking, and resolves emotional sensitivity along with any physical sensitivity.

The Planetary Qualities of Hypericum perforatum

St. John's wort has a strong relationship to the sun. Cases of Seasonal Affective Disorder (SAD; associated with winter depression) respond well to *Hypericum perforatum*. In mythic and alchemical terms, the sun relates to the Father, and the person needing St John's wort may have some relationship problems, whether real or imagined, with either the literal father or with some authority figure. The person may dream of a father figure. Yet this association can also relate to the "father" of the self—the leadership and authority of the personality—which may be weak, thereby causing depression. *Hypericum perforatum* enables the individual to take charge of life, providing him with the energy and will to prosecute his own interests.

The sun relates to the solar plexus, a complex ganglion of nerves in the center of the body. Here, "undigested" emotions can play havoc with actual digestion and assimilation of food. For sensitive people who cannot digest their emotions and who then manifest these problems in nervous ailments—headaches, pains, and a variety of digestive complaints—St. John's wort enables them to process their fears, thereby reducing anxiety.

Combinations

St. John's wort combines well with *Calendula officinalis* for wounds and as a mouthwash for dental surgery and periodontitis. They can be added to aqueous cream and used on the skin.

Contraindications

Sun allergy has been found in some animals that eat the plant, but in humans, external treatment with *Hypericum perforatum* oil, made by infusing the flowers in olive oil, seems to enable sun tolerance.

There may be some adverse reactions with pharmaceutical drugs. Those taking prescription drugs should consult their medical advisor before embarking on treatment with spagyric essence of St. John's wort.

Iris versicolor

Iridaceae

Common name: Iris

Other common names: Blue flag, wild iris. The plant is known in French as *iris;* in German, *Blaue Iris;* in Italian, *giglio azzura;* in Spanish, *mavi.*

Ruling planet: Jupiter

Parts used: Roots

The Plant

The Iridaceae family, comprising eighteen hundred species across the world, flourishes in both tropical and temperate climates, but particularly in Central America and South America, South Africa, and the Mediterranean basin. It is related to the lily family, Liliaceae.

Several plants in the Iridaceae family are known to have medicinal uses. These include *Iris fetidissima* (headaches and hernias), *Iris florentina* (oris root; delirium), *Iris germanica* (dropsy), and *Iris tenax* (pains in the ileocecal region, appendicitis). *Crocus sativus* (saffron) belongs to this family too, as do freesia and gladiolus, but the chief therapeutic plant in this family is *Iris versicolor.* The dried root (rhizome) is the part used.

Native to North America and with a long therapeutic history among the Native Americans, iris was also taken up by early settlers and earned a place in eclectic medicine. It grows best in peaty soils that are fairly damp. A perennial, it has thick-branched rhizome root stock from which stout, coarse stems emerge. Leaves are sword-shaped. The flowers, appearing in early or mid-summer, are usually blue or violet streaked with yellow, or white with purple veins.

In Greek mythology, Iris was a messenger between heaven and earth, the sea and the underworld—a feminine counterpart to Hermes. Iris is the personification of the rainbow, also a message of the divine on earth in both ancient Greek myths and in the Old Testament, in which a rainbow is sent as a promise to Noah that the earth would never again be subject to flood. The flower is named after the rainbow because of the wide variety of colors it can exhibit—indicated by the name *versicolor.* When we look at how the plant grows—its roots in bogs or marshes, but nonetheless reaching, erect and tall, to the sky—the iris seems to embody aspiration and spiritual longing. As the *fleur de lys,* it was the emblem of French kings. The upright stem and flower resemble a scepter, and the three main petals of the fleur de lys were thought to symbolize faith, wisdom, and valor.

Sphere of Therapeutic Action

Used by both the Greeks and Romans, iris has a long medicinal history, but it is perhaps the North American Indians who held it in highest regard for its therapeutic qualities. They used the roots for poultices to treat rheumatism, ulcers, sores, wounds, and bruises. Although iris was dropped from the U.S. Official Pharmacopoeia in 1938, its herbal use may be due for a revival in view of the rapid rise of diabetes in the developed world. Iris has long been thought to have an affinity with the pancreas and to be a specific of hypoglycemic conditions, which are often a precursor to migraines. In India, iris has been used to treat obesity, because the root has an effect on fat catabolism.

Major glands are the province of this remedy: chiefly the pancreas, the thyroid, the liver, and gallbladder, as well as mucous membranes of the gastric tract and the salivary glands. In those who may benefit from iris, the abdomen may be sore, with pains in the liver or burning pains in the pancreas. The pains of the gut, whether of the throat, esophagus, or stomach, may be burning or cutting. The tongue may feel as though scalded, and there is a greasy or sweet taste in the mouth and copious saliva, especially during a period of headache. Stools may be loose, but can burn like fire. There is acidity in the stomach, as though the contents of the stomach have turned to vinegar, and a strange characteristic is that the sweat may also smell of vinegar.

Iris can be used to treat sinusitis, eye problems, and headaches or even migraines with stomach disturbances. The sick headaches or migraines may be periodic—weekly or fortnightly—and they may come on after mental strain and exhaustion. Iris problems often manifest on weekends or when the person feels he can begin to relax. The first sign of an impending headache may be blurred vision, the sensation of a weight on the neck, or gastric upset. The cause is usually stress or overwork. Iris helps to regularize intestinal function, reducing gastric acidity, stimulating the flow of bile, and normalizing liver function.

The Salt Qualities of Iris versicolor

Iris is high in chromium, which has been found to help in fat metabolism, as well as magnesium and calcium. In addition to tannins, the root contains 2.5 percent acrid resins with traces of salicylic acid and phenolic glycosides that act upon the parasympathetic nervous system. These help to produce saliva, sweat, and bile, all of which help to normalize the system. Iridin, another glycoside, is a diuretic.

The Sulphur-Soul Qualities of Iris versicolor

The volatile oils contained in the iris root taste slightly sweet and give off a mild aromatic scent. The iris flower that raises its lovely blooms high above the mud in which it grows is symbolic of the iris personality. Physically, iris people may be tall and slender, attractive, even beautiful, and may give the impression of being delicate. Artistic and charming, they are good at hiding their own insecurities and unhappiness. They may in fact be depressives, struggling with addictions and abusive relationships and having troubling dreams of corpses and graves. The flower holds up its head to the heavens, but the person feels a weight upon his neck that bows him down as though he is overburdened. There may be headaches, even migraines, especially on days off. While something is expected of them, they struggle to rise above whatever pulls them down, whether a difficult situation at home or even just a sense that the world is a difficult and evil place. When they are by themselves, however, they succumb to the headaches or to tears.

The Planetary Qualities of Iris versicolor

The liver is ruled by Jupiter, the planet of expansion and acquisitiveness. The Jupiter individual may be covetous and consume with the eyes, wanting more than he needs, whether possessions or food or experiences. These individuals exhibit a desire to collect the world, like the tourist who snaps a picture of a famous monument and then rushes on to the next, not taking the time to enjoy the actual experience of beauty. The person may put more food on his plate than is good to eat, and biliousness may be a key physical symptom. The desire is really for spiritual growth, but, just as the iris is literally "bogged down," he may be tethered to materialism—that is, the person will go on acquiring material possessions. Unable to lift themselves, there may be an element of self-disgust, and they may be unable to laugh at themselves. Worried, troubled, anxious, they need to take the wider view. In the negative state, a troubled liver, low spirits, despondency, and low stamina are all typical of those needing this remedy. Taken over time, the face will become clear and the eyes more radiant as the individual begins to realize his true spiritual self.

Combinations

Iris and St. John's wort can be taken together if the symptoms fit the need for both and the individual wants to make changes in his or her life.

Contraindications

Sensitive people may find that handling the plants produces contact dermatitis. *All parts of the plant may be harmful if ingested.* Only the root is used medicinally.

Melissa officinalis

Lamiaceae
Common name: Lemon balm
Other names: In French, the plant is known as *citronelle;* in German, *Zitronen-melisse;* in Italian, *cedronella;* in Spanish, *erba cedrata.*

Ruling planets: Moon and Mercury; according to Culpeper, Jupiter in Cancer

Parts used: Leaves picked before the plant flowers

The Plant

Native to the Mediterranean, this plant grows widely across Europe and North Africa and is naturalized in North America and other parts of the world. This perennial plant likes a sunny position and protection from frost. Its stems are square and slightly hairy. The ovate leaves grow opposite and are crenate-dentate. The leaves are pale yellow-green or bright green, and small white flowers appear on the plant in the early autumn. As the name implies, it is a plant loved by bees; the Greeks called it *melissophyllon,* or "bee leaf."

If possible, consider using only fresh leaves for your spagyric remedy, because this herb soon loses its wonderful fragrance when dried, and its therapeutic powers are diminished in long-term storage.

Sphere of Therapeutic Action

Arabs noticed that this plant has the power to lift depression. Avicenna recommended lemon balm as a heart tonic, a plant to make the heart merry. For Paracelsus, it was a true elixir of life. It is useful as an immune stimulant against colds and flu. Hot infusions induce sweating to reduce a fever. As a sedative, it soothes the nerves, ameliorates headache and depression, calms restlessness, and eases digestion after meals. It has widespread use to strengthen the nerves against stress and strain, and it has been said to protect the cerebrum of the brain and to be an effective treatment for autonomic disorders—equaling modern tranquilizers in this respect. Those who may be treated with lemon balm may have palpitations due to nervous anxiety and depression. Both Pliny and Galen recognized its ability to heal sores, bites, and stings. Fresh leaves can be used externally on sores and insect bites.

For centuries *Melissa officinalis* has been regarded as an aid to digestion, for which purpose it is sometimes added to vinegars and liqueurs.

It is an ingredient in fine liqueurs such as Benedictine and Chartreuse. Relaxing and rejuvenating, the essence works on the disturbed nervous system and the digestive problems associated with nervous tension and anxiety.

Emotions play a vital role in all our physiological systems, stimulating appropriate secretions in the body, especially in the digestive tract. If we eat when we are stressed or unhappy, the food is hard to digest. It is not surprising, therefore, to find that *Melissa officinalis* has sedative and digestive effects. It also assists in the peripheral blood circulatory system, reducing spasm and lifting headaches. When we feel loved and loving, we experience relaxation of the spirit, and even the veins and arteries relax. As the blood vessels relax and dilate, the blood moves more freely and circulation is improved.

The Salt Qualities of Melissa officinalis

The essential oil contains citral, linalool, citronellal, and geraniol, as well as tannins, resin, rosmarinic, and succinic acid. This calming, sedative herb is antiviral and antibacterial and helps to lower fevers. Clinical trials and laboratory studies have shown *Melissa officinalis* to be effective for herpes (both *Herpes simplex* and *Herpes zoster*) because of its ability to block receptors used by the virus for cell adsorption, preventing viral entry into the cells and thereby blocking viral replication.

The Sulphur-Soul Qualities of Melissa officinalis

Lemon balm is said to have a very high vibrational level, and it brings the spiritual support of heavenly forces into those who are listless and discouraged by the shape their lives are taking. Culpeper recommended *Melissa officinalis* for the person who is fearful and so timid that she cannot fight her own corner. She will not stand up for herself, nor can she be roused to a healthy and appropriate degree of anger. Instead, she puts up with everything in a resigned way. Culpeper classified lemon balm as a "hardening medicine," one that corrects a tendency to dampness and susceptibility to infections on the physical plane, as well as hardening the weak will in the psychological sphere. Lemon balm is a plant that goes directly to the heart of the problem of existence, the existential fears concerning the present and the future. Thus it is possible to distinguish plant energies depending on whether the individual has issues of the past (hawthorn) or of the present and future (lemon balm).

The Planetary Qualities of Melissa officinalis

The Moon rules the brain, stomach, and digestion. In melissa the memory, nervous energy, and will power all need to be strengthened to deal with the challenges of life. There may be low spirits; John Evelyn comments that melissa is "sovereign for the brain. It strengthens the memory and powerfully chases away melancholy." The lovely, lemon-scented oil is indeed pleasant, soothing, and uplifting. Mercury governs anxiety and nervous disorders.

Contraindications

This is a hypotensive, so care should be taken with people who are taking heart medication. In addition, it may inhibit thyroid activity.

Rosmarinus officinalis

Lamiaceae
Common name: Rosemary
Other names: In French, the plant is known as *encensier;* in German, *Rosmarin;* in Italian, *rosemarine;* in Spanish, *romere.*
Ruling planet: Sun; Sun in Aries (Culpeper)
Parts used: Dried leaves or fresh leaves and flowers

The Plant

Rosemary is indigenous to the Mediterranean basin, including Portugal, Spain, France, Italy, Cypress, Turkey, Greece and the Aegean islands, the coast of North Africa, and the Canary Islands. With its versatility and utility in both culinary and medicinal use, it has been widely cultivated elsewhere. Provided it is not subjected to too much cold or damp, it is an adaptable plant of bushy habit. It is an evergreen perennial shrub with strongly aromatic leaves. The springy stems become woody as the plant ages. Leaves are simple and slightly leathery and they grow opposite. The flowers are mostly blue and grow in short racemes.

The therapeutic history of rosemary goes back to antiquity in Greek medicine and to Egyptian funeral rites. The powers of regeneration attributed to this sacred plant led the ancient Egyptians to place bushes in tombs with the dead. Its antiseptic properties have given rise to its use as a fumigant: In the medieval period there was a tradition of burning it on fires in hospitals to cleanse the air while also lifting the mood of patients.

Sphere of Therapeutic Action

Blood circulation is the special sphere of this plant. It is ideal for those ailments caused by inadequate or disturbed circulation, whether to the brain or to the heart. Headaches or even migraines can be ameliorated, especially those caused by stress or digestive upset. As an antispasmodic, it relieves migraines by dilating the cerebral vascular tissue. If there is exhaustion or brain fog, poor memory, low blood pressure, lethargy, and pessimism—when the fires of life burn low—rosemary brings clarity and energy. Its rousing qualities make it a valuable herb in the management of myalgic encephalopathy (ME) and chronic fatigue, but it should be used with caution and gentleness if there is long-standing fatigue. The rousing properties of rosemary may exhaust in the long-term if an individual has insufficient underlying vitality to cope with additional stimulation. On the other hand, if an individual needs concentration to work intensively for short periods, rosemary helps with mental steadiness, and it sharpens the memory.

Culpeper advocated its use when the pulse was soft and slow and the person was weak both in body and will. In terms of the four humors, rosemary is characteristic of the phlegmatic type—those who are typically cold and moist. Culpeper also classified rosemary as one of his *arthriticals,* a term he used for medicines for joints. Used topically as an oil on the skin, rosemary draws blood to the surface, increasing heat locally in the tissues, which helps to relieve the pain of rheumatism.

Rosemary essential oil is often added to topical beauty products for the skin for the same reason. It draws the blood supply to the skin and helps in the absorption of constituents of oils or creams. For its power of drawing heat to the body, rosemary is valuable in the instance of chills—that is, when a person is extremely cold, particularly in the extremities, and has no inner warmth or thirst. As a nerve stimulant, it energizes and enlivens the brain and nervous system. Taking the spagyric essence helps to clarify and beautify the complexion (but beware of the contraindications, listed below).

The Salt Qualities of **Rosmarinus officinalis**

New research confirms the age-old wisdom that rosemary offers major neuroprotective benefits without the disturbances associated with drugs. Drugs that help in neurodegenerative disorders also tend to interfere with the normal function of the nervous system. Yet rosemary improves brain function without damaging its delicate processes. Constituents of rosemary include selenium, an excellent antioxidant that makes rosemary ideal for premature aging. Selenium strengthens the cardiovascular system and primes both red and white blood cells. Research has found a definite correlation between low levels of selenium and a high incidence of cancer. In addition, hydrogen, the most widespread constituent of the universe, is very high in this plant. Sixty-three percent of human atoms are hydrogen, and a similar proportion of seawater is atomically hydrogen. Rosemary also contains calcium, iron, and vitamin B_6 (pyridoxine), which assists the formation of healthy red blood cells and the production of adrenalin, insulin, and antibodies. Pyridoxine also assists the metabolism of protein, fats, and carbohydrates. A deficiency of this vitamin has been noted in premenstrual tension. As well as rosmarinic acid, rosemary also contains carnosal and carnosic acid, which are powerful neuroprotective agents known for scavenging peroxyl and hydroxyl radicals.

The Sulphur-Soul Qualities of Rosmarinus officinalis

Rosemary is highly stimulating and is excellent for the circulatory system and mental acuity. As Shakespeare noted, it enhances the memory. Rosemary may also lead the memory to recollection of who we really are on a spiritual level. Just as it helps to lift the spirits in depression, it also lifts the spirits in a religious sense. For centuries it has been used as a votive scent in the Greek Orthodox Church. Its regular use brings confidence in one's path in life, purification of intention, stability, and perseverance in rising to meet one's long-term life purpose.

The Planetary Qualities of Rosmarinus officinalis

As Culpeper noted, rosemary comes into flower when the sun is in Aries. This astrological sign also rules the head in zodiacal anatomy, and rosemary has a particular affinity for the head, because it is stimulating to the memory. The plant is also sometimes classified under the dominion of the moon, which has affinities with the brain, memory, beliefs, awareness, and receptivity.

Contraindications

Always carefully evaluate each person's circumstances before giving rosemary, because its stimulating effects can be harmful. It should be avoided in patients with any history of epilepsy or high blood pressure. Avoid use in pregnancy. Never ingest essential oils by themselves. When indicated, give rosemary in small doses, and always dilute the spagyric essence well. Dose: five drops in a small glass of water. A few drops may also be added to a fine, light white wine or used to flavor honey.

Salvia officinalis

Lamiaceae

Common name: Sage

Other common names: Red sage. This plant is known in French as *sauge;* in German, *Salbei;* in Italian, *salvia grande;* and in Spanish, *salvia.*

Ruling planets: Moon and Mercury
Parts used: Leaves picked just before flowering and in the early fall

The Plant

Sage is a perennial herb that grows to a height of eighteen inches. It is indigenous to southern Europe and to North America. The leaves, which are opposite, are long oblong-lanceolate or ovate and grow to between one and four inches long. The upper surface of the leaves is a downy gray-green, with a depressed mid-rib and veins. Blue flowers appear in whorls in June and July.

New research focuses on the potential for sage extracts as a treatment for Alzheimer's disease. To the Romans, however, who regarded sage as a sacred plant, it was not used as an herb for old age but for the beginning of life: it was thought to help women conceive. Romans took it for its toning properties, whatever their age. North American Indians have also revered this plant as sacred, and they used it for spiritual purposes. In spiritual practice around the world, it is burned at religious ceremonies, and water infused with the herb is used for purification and bathing.

Sphere of Therapeutic Action

Salvia officinalis was perhaps the most important therapeutic herb of medieval Europe. Despite its long therapeutic history, reaching back to the ancient Greeks, this herb has been rather overlooked as a medicine in modern times. Yet as drug-resistant tuberculosis is making a comeback, and because a relatively high proportion of the population of many Western countries is now in the older age group, its medicinal properties are worth reconsidering. It is an ideal gentle medicine for the aged and has been called the longevity herb. Gerard comments: "Sage is singularly good for the head and brain; it quickeneth the senses and memory, strengtheneth the sinews, restoreth health to those that have palsy and taketh away shaky trembling of the members."[8]

Salvia officinalis has been known as a treatment for symptoms of depression, poor memory, mental confusion, anxiety, and nervousness.

Also, it is a treatment for vertigo and headaches, particularly those of older people. It is specific for ailments of the respiratory system: it is used to treat sore throats; tonsillitis; inflammation of the mouth, gums, and throat; laryngitis; and pharyngitis. It is also a specific for nightsweats of those suffering from respiratory disorders. Asthma sufferers may obtain relief from its antispasm capacity. Sage is also of value in treating loss of appetite and a weak stomach. It acts as a digestive, reducing flatulence and gastrointestinal catarrh. It reduces high levels of blood sugar in diabetes. In women, it can be helpful for diminishing the hot flashes of menopause, and it slows breast milk production when a child is being weaned.

The Salt Qualities of Salvia officinalis

Constituents of sage include camphor, a transparent or waxy substance with a characteristic odor that stimulates the intellectual faculties and soothes nervous excitement. Camphor is also known medicinally as a treatment for respiratory oppression and blocked noses. Research has found in sage some twenty-three terpenoids with antioxidant effects; Vitamins A, B complex, and C; calcium; and potassium. Among sage's other constituents are ten phenolic compounds, cineole, borneol, pinene, salvene esters, and sesquiterpenes. Thujone, found in sage, is a powerful antiseptic and antibiotic, meaning it is suitable for gingivitis, dental abscesses, gum decay, mouth ulcers, and all throat infections. Thujone is also a vermifuge. Phenolic acid is specific against *Staphylococcus aureus*. The ash content of sage can be 8 percent.

The Sulphur-Soul Qualities of Salvia officinalis

Always considered a sacred plant, the herb of salvation, sage cleanses and purifies the spirit. It helps to integrate the spiritual into life. It preserves the light of reason, memory, and creative thought in old age. An herb for the first and the last stages of life, sage calls the powers of heaven into the human world as a plant that opens the spirit to conceive new life and gracefully prepares the spirit for its final journey.

The Planetary Qualities of Salvia officinalis

Sage is a remedy of the fifth chakra—the throat chakra. The throat and respiratory organs come under the dominion of Mercury, and the moon governs the brain and memory. In addition to healing the lungs and throat, Mercury also governs active intelligence, analytical intellect, and reasoning powers. The moon represents awareness, sensitivity, receptivity, memory, and imagination. Speech, writing, and communication are Hermetic gifts found in teachers, speakers, actors, and singers—all of whom suffer one time or another from throat problems due to inhibition of the fifth chakra, or they suffer simply from overuse of the voice. In individuals, the influence of Mercury helps to bring a sense of rational balance to the moon propensity for suspicious, instinctive, confused behavior. With the positive gifts of imagination, memory, and sympathy, the moon balances Mercury's tendency toward impatience, criticism, and overrationality.

Contraindications

Avoid its use for those who have high blood pressure, blood in the urine, pregnancy, or epilepsy.

Sambucus nigra

Caprifoliaceae
Common name: Elderflower
Other common names: Black elder, elder. It is known in French as *sureau;* in German, *Holunder;* in Italian, *sambreo;* in Spanish, *sauco.*
Ruling Planet: Mercury
Parts used: Elderflowers, bark, or berries for use in tinctures (each has its own sphere of action). Berries, which are full of vitamin C and are believed to ward off winter colds and flu, can be used to make cordials or wine. The berries of true *Sambuccus nigra* are not considered poisonous, but the berries of some other varieties of elder may be. Leaves can be poisonous and should be avoided.

The Plant

Caprifoliaceae is the botanical classification of the Honeysuckle family, which is widespread in North America, East Asia, and across the northern temperate regions. Elderflower tolerates shade and poor soil and will grow on waste ground. A quick-grower, wind-resistant and hardy, it is an ideal plant to use when establishing a framework for other plantings in adverse conditions. The North American native plant is *Sambucus canadensis,* but the slightly larger European *Sambucus nigra* is widely naturalized, and both share similar chemistry. Take care to use the right plant: the North American *S. racemosa,* which has red berries, should not be used: the berries can be toxic. In addition, there is a Dwarf Elder *S. Ebulus,* which is also another species. *Sambucus nigra* is a plant widely distributed around the world.

There is a number of folkloric myths and legends about this plant that have persisted through the centuries. Most of these superstitions concern fright. Even today, some hedgecutters don't like to disturb the elder, for the legends tell of spirits of the tree that might pursue them. The elder has long been associated with the cross of Christ and the Judas tree. In Scandinavia there are myths about the Hylde-Moer, the elder-tree mother who lives in the tree and punishes those who cut it.

Sphere of Therapeutic Action

This plant has a particular affinity for the lungs and kidneys. It is a powerful cleanser, acting on the respiratory and urinary systems and the skin. A keynote indication is when an individual sleeps into an attack, waking suddenly with mental anxiety, asthma, dyspnea, or perspiration. The person may have dreamed of suffocation and then awakened to find themselves in a suffocative attack. Though the elderberry is used for bronchitis, asthma, and other respiratory difficulties, including colds and flu, elderflowers are used medicinally for acne, eczema, psoriasis, and burns. As a beautifier, water distilled from the flowers has been used for centuries as an eyewash and a gentle skin lotion that soothes dry skin and relieves sunburn.

The inner part of the bark also has therapeutic uses as a diuretic, purgative, and, in larger doses, as an emetic. The leaves also have diuretic and purgative properties and can be used to make an expectorant or to reduce bleeding.

The Salt Qualities of Sambucus nigra

The plant is extraordinarily rich in nutrients. The berries contain the vitamins A, B, and C; iron, calcium, and potassium. The leaves contain hydrocyanic acid and potassium nitrate and can be toxic. These substances affect the respiratory organs, heart, and blood vessels. Elder has a powerful affinity for the kidneys and is almost a specific for nephritis and the rapid onset of dropsy. In common with hawthorn, the elder contains cyanogenic glycosides that are antispasmodic and sedative. They calm the heart rate and improve digestion.

The Sulphur-Soul Qualities of Sambucus nigra

Individuals who are easily frightened or those who have a history of fright will benefit from this plant. The person in need of the remedy may visibly tremble. Sometimes the fright has a close connection to losing a parent (usually a mother) at a very early age. In *Cymbeline*, Shakespeare mentions the tree as a symbol of grief. Both asthma—holding on to the breath—and edema—holding on to water in the body—represent the psychological need to hold on to something very dear, and both are a somatization of the deep fear occasioned by sudden loss. As a result of trauma, there may be delusions and dreams with visions of horrible faces.

The elder essence helps individuals to mature into their own independence and realize that a parent cannot always be available to take care of them. It allows them to shape their own lives, making decisions for themselves, and to accept that in the great mysteries of life and death, we cannot always know why someone lives and another does not. Lives can become stuck if there is too much fear. The essence works on the fourth chakra, the heart, and reminds us that love drives out fear.

The essence also works on the fifth chakra, the throat and lungs. Fear stifles the breath. Articulating fears may help individuals to come to understanding.

Planetary Qualities of Sambucus nigra

All respiratory diseases come under the dominion of Mercury, the messenger, which governs the relationship between the inner and the outer being, The lungs are a frontier between life forces in the outer world and the inner body, where the breath, oxygen, *prana,* chi is processed. In breathing, we take in air from the outside, and, having processed it for our benefit, we breathe it out again. It is a vital exchange between the inner body and the outer world that is normally effortless and requires no thought. Anxiety and fear can interrupt this process, bringing on the kind of asthmatic attacks typical of the *Sambucus nigra* state of fear, which are characteristically expressed as an inability to expire. Afflicted individuals hold on to the breath so that the lungs do not empty sufficiently to draw in another breath, hence the feeling of suffocation. This sets up a vicious circle in which fear interrupts the normal breathing cycle, producing sensations of suffocation, when the individual literally fears for his life. Those in this state must learn the art of letting go, a process of coming to trust the universe and their own responses to it. The skin is another organ in which the inner and outer world meet. Asthma and skin ailments can often alternate: if eczema is suppressed with steroids, the person may develop asthma, forming another vicious cycle.

Combination

Elderflower essence works well with yarrow.

Contraindications

Do not eat the leaves or berries raw. Always cook the berries in a little water before using them. In culinary use, they can be added *in small quantities* to other stewed fruits, such as apples for puddings.

Taraxacum officinale

Asteraceae

Common name: Dandelion

Other names: In French, it is called *dent de lion,* from which the English name derives. In Latin, it is *dens leonis;* in German, *Löwenzahn;* in Italian, *dente de leone;* in Spanish, *diente de leon.*

Ruling planet: Jupiter

Parts used: Leaves or roots or leaves and roots together

The Plant

One of the most common members of the Asteraceae family is the dandelion, which is widespread in the northern hemisphere. A plant thought to be thirty million years old, *Taraxacum officinale* tolerates a wide variety of soils and, in an optimum environment, may flower almost all year round.

In many European languages, it is commonly referred to as lion's teeth, to which the serrated edges of the leaves have been likened.

What appears to be a single flower in the dandelion is in fact many ray florets gathered onto a single hollow, hairless stalk. Each petal is a flower that will produce a seed, giving rise to the wonderful gossamer seed heads so characteristic of this plant. The single taproot is surmounted by a rosette of leaves above ground, from which the single central stalk emerges. When the flowers wither, the emerging seed head is also a wonder of plant engineering: a spherical "clock" of single-seeded fruits, each with fine hairs that enable wind dispersal over long distances. The spagyric essence is made of the whole plant—flowers, leaves, and root together.

Sphere of Therapeutic Action

The yellow color of the dandelion flower is associated with the liver (per the doctrine of signatures), which is its traditional sphere of therapeutic action. The planet ruler of *Taraxacum officinale* is Jupiter, the largest planet, just as the liver is the largest internal organ in the body.

At least since the Middle Ages, the dandelion plant has been used as a diuretic in the treatment of liver and kidney disorders. Unlike modern pharmaceutical diuretics, however, *Taraxacum officinale* naturally contains a high proportion of potassium. It is therefore safe to take as a cleanser of the liver, gallbladder, spleen, and the urinary system, and it has proved useful in cancer of the bladder. It gently promotes bowel regularity where there is chronic, stubborn constipation due to liver derangement. In those who may benefit from this remedy, there may be pain and heaviness or a sensation of fullness in the region of both the liver and spleen, with or without jaundice (yellowing of skin). Headaches may be violent and right-sided, typical of liver disturbance.

Symptoms of liver disturbance may also involve skin ailments; joint pains; blurred eyesight; and digestive complaints, especially chronic constipation or yellowish diarrhea. Additionally, there may be a general torpor and fatigue often accompanied by anemia and extreme sensitivity to cold. The individual will crave warm food and drinks and may be sleepy by day, especially after meals, but insomnia is common. When an individual wakes in the small hours, between one and four in the morning, and is unable to fall asleep again, a liver disturbance is a possible cause. In the nighttime hours, the liver is at its most active, cleansing and detoxifying and processing the day's intake of nourishment. We can note that the flowers of *Taraxacum officinale* do not open to the moon and stars, but rather in the morning, and they close up again as dusk appears.

When someone has allergies, the overall physical constitution must be supported, and a combination of herbs chosen to improve immune competence will be enhanced by the addition of *Taraxacum officinale*. Fat and sugar metabolism are also the province of the liver, and there is growing evidence that it is the liver, more than the pancreas, which is implicated in type 2 diabetes mellitus.[9] Certainly, optimal liver function is critical to health and energy, and dandelion is an excellent remedy for liver support in cases of type 2 diabetes mellitus.

The Salt Qualities of Taraxacum officinale

Dandelion is extraordinarily rich in nutrients, vitamins, and minerals. Fluorine helps the production of strong bones and teeth, and iron helps the body to make good-quality blood. Manganese, potassium, sodium, and silica assist in bladder and kidney problems and cardiac arrhythmias with water retention. Magnesium is said to aid problems with obesity and constipation, and chromium helps to reduce cholesterol and obesity. Regular courses of treatment with dandelion essence may be particularly useful for prediabetics. The leaves are high in vitamins A and C.

The Sulphur-Soul Qualities of Taraxacum officinale

There is a theme of bitterness running through the dandelion picture. The leaves of the plant, often used in salads, taste bitter, rather like chicory. The person who may benefit from dandelion may report a bitter taste in the mouth and may indicate that the sputum tastes sour. Life may taste bitter too: the person may be in a gloomy mood, depressive and indolent and easily irritated. He may be reluctant to get to work, but he performs conscientiously when he does work. The bitter person may "bite"—that is, fly off the handle with sudden anger.

The liver is a patient organ, putting up with a considerable amount of toxic abuse from incorrect diet, alcohol, and drugs, without complaint. It is a silent organ, too, emitting few complaints of pain or discomfort until pathology is somewhat advanced. Yet in the mental realm, the person needing *Taraxacum officinale* may be irritable and "liverish," and inclined to "vent his spleen" when the occasion arises. In the Chinese five-element system of medicine, the liver is associated with the noise of shouting.

The Planetary Qualities of Taraxacum officinale

Jupiter, the planet that rules the plant and the liver, is the planet of expansiveness. It is a planet associated with growth and opportunity. The sight of dandelions in the countryside raises the spirits; with its cheerful, bright yellow flowers, the dandelion radiates joy in life. This is what the spagyric essence of *Taraxacum officinale* can do: bring an opening to life, freeing the individual of anger and bitterness. As the liver is soothed, cleansed, and refreshed, the person's anger and revolt are calmed and transformed into love and joy. From being tired, lethargic, and easily irritated, the person regains vitality, a good temper, and a true sense of *joie de vivre*.

Contraindications

Liver cleansing can occasionally have unwelcome effects, especially when a liver imbalance gives rise to skin ailments. If the liver is extremely toxic, nausea may result. In such a case, start treatment at a much lower dose and build up gradually as the liver improves.

Urtica dioica

Urticaceae
Common name: Greater stinging nettle
Other names: The plant is known in French as *grande ortie;* in German, *Grosse Brandnetel;* in Italian, *grande ortica;* in Spanish, *ortiga.*
Ruling planet: Mars
Parts used: Leaf and root

The Plant

Greater stinging nettle is widely distributed across the world, and in fact, there are several medicinal nettles: *U. urens,* lesser stinging nettle, is used in homeopathy, while *U. dioica* is used in medical herbalism. The two have similar therapeutic uses and are sometimes said to be interchangeable for medicinal purposes. The leaves of nettle are ovate and toothed, with tiny hairs, each one of which can inject formic acid into the skin, causing a painful, red rash. It is worth persevering, though, because nettles pack a real punch both as a food and a medicine. They punch above their weight in vitamins and minerals, so no wonder nettles have been called the most useful of all herbs. Free to all—because no one covets them—they grow wild in abundance and are a natural, high-quality vitamin and mineral supplement. The plant stings only when fresh.

Known as *wergulu* to the Anglo-Saxons, nettles were regarded as a sacred plant. Nettles are one of the five bitter herbs to be eaten at the Jewish festival of Passover. Nettles stay the course: they are almost impossible to eradicate or subdue. They are activators, vitalizing other plants and stimulating growth. Thus they are an excellent companion plant, especially for herbs. They seem to promote the essential oil content in nearby plants as well as encouraging the growth of strawberries. Animals eat them for their nourishing and healing powers, and several species of Lepidoptera rely on them for food. As an ecology plant, nettle is remarkable for its ability to process and remove toxic pollutants from the earth and air. It is often seen growing over waste ground or along roadsides. Obviously, with nettles' abilities to absorb toxins, it is very important to choose a healthy environment from which to harvest your plants.

Nettles can be picked from early spring through summer to autumn. Use ceramic scissors to cut the tops, and lift them into your basket. They can be used fresh or dried and can be frozen without too much loss of nourishment.

Nettle roots can be dug up as required, but these are best in the autumn. Wash them well and dry them on a cake rack or screen. When ready, they should be brittle and should break cleanly.

When you prepare the spagyric essence, some of the minerals in nettles are not extracted by alcohol, so it will be necessary to prepare a half quantity using the alcohol maceration method described on page 102 and prepare the other half by making an infusion. When your alcohol tincture is ready, make the infusion by pouring 2 pints (1 liter) of boiled filtered water over 1 ounce of dried herb. Cover and leave to stand for several hours or overnight. Strain carefully through coffee filter papers or muslin. Add the infusion to the tincture, but make sure that you have more alcohol tincture than water-based infusion for preserving purposes.

Sphere of Therapeutic Action

Gerard comments that Pliny said the oil from the stinging nettle would take away the pain of being stung by the nettle. Nettles do indeed contain histamines—a perfect example of the homeopathic principle in action. Recent research shows that nettle is an effective analgesic in rheumatism, reducing pain and disability (more often than placebo) and improving the quality of sleep. Nettle promotes elimination of urine, nourishes the blood in anemia, removes blood sugar, and supports treatment for diabetes. In mild type 2 diabetes, which can be controlled by diet alone, it is an excellent year-round support. Nettle stimulates the circulation by causing the dilation of the peripheral blood vessels and thus making the process more efficient. With its deep cleansing powers, it stimulates epithelial cells in the skin, enabling them to release accretions from the environment. Its action is centrifugal, cleansing from within to without, from the bones to the skin. With regular use, it helps to restructure the physical body. Nettle strengthens the nervous system against environmental influence and protects it from stress. It also protects the organism from disturbances of electromagnetic fields.

As an amphoteric, nettle helps to regularize the flow of milk. (It promotes milk production if scanty, and reduces production if it is excessive.) Cows fed on nettles have enhanced milk production. Nettle action is diuretic, but it is also regulatory: it has been found to diminish the frequency of nighttime urination in men with benign prostatic hyperplasia.

The Salt Qualities of Urtica dioica

Nettles have high levels of protein, more than any other commonly used plant, and high levels of chlorophyll, a substance common to most plants. Chlorophyll enables photosynthesis and gives plants their green color; it stores the energy of the sun. Chlorophyll is to the plant what blood is to the human being, and both blood and chlorophyll depend upon iron for their metabolic processes. Iron acts as a catalyst that speeds up reaction, helping to promote granulation of tissue in wound healing. With its high iron content, nettle is wonderful for making good-quality blood and is ideal for iron-deficiency anemia. It also removes sugar and toxins from the blood and enhances the effects of vitamins and minerals. With calcium, silica, manganese, and sulfur as additional constituents, nettle assists in building strong bones and in tissue building and wound healing. Other constituents include acetylcholine, a neurotransmitter utilized in the central and peripheral nervous systems. With high levels of vitamins C and A, it is a tremendous immunity booster.

The Sulphur-Soul Qualities of Urtica dioica

Nettle has rousing, rejuvenating, and resurrecting powers on the weakened individual. With its strong nutritional and regularizing properties, nettle enables the strengthening of all parts of the human being, not only the physical body. It brings qualities of courage and idealism, and strengthens will power. In a positive nettle state, the individual exhibits passion and enthusiasm, independence of thought and action, and the ability to seize the initiative. In a community, such people will demonstrate leadership abilities, stimulating and inspiring others with their enthusiasm.

The Planetary Qualities of Urtica dioica

Culpeper comments:

> This is also an herb Mars claims dominion over. You know Mars is hot and dry, and you know as well that Winter is cold and moist; then you may know as well the reason why Nettle-tops eaten in the spring consume the phlegmatic superfluities in the body of man, that the coldness and moistness of winter hath left behind. The roots or leaves boiled, or the juice of either of them, or both made into an electuary with honey and sugar is a safe and sure medicine to open

the pipes and passages of the lungs, which is the cause of wheezing and shortness of breath, and helps to expectorate tough phlegm, as also to raise the imposthumed pleurisy.[10]

The Mars qualities of nettle bring vitality and courage. Mars, the god of war, ruler of the blood, brings energy and assertive qualities to the physical being, strengthening all systems. Iron is the planetary metal of Mars and is essential to correct anemia and to help energize and purify the blood. When the physical body is strengthened, the personality is more courageous, daring to act, daring to speak out against injustice, and putting words into action.

Combinations
Nettle can be combined with yarrow or elderflower.

Contraindications
The upper leaves provide excellent nourishment, ideal for use during pregnancy, but avoid the roots when pregnant.

Notes

Introduction: The Healing Art of Spagyric Medicine

1. CDC website, www.cdc.gov (accessed December 1, 2009).

Chapter 1. A Brief History of Alchemy

1. Antoine Faivre, *The Eternal Hermes: From Greek God to Alchemical Magus* (Grand Rapids, Mich.: Phanes Press, 1995), 18–20.
2. *Corpus Hermeticum,* Book V:10, in Clement Salaman, Dorine van Oyen, William D. Wharton, trans., *The Way of Hermes* (London: Duckworth, 1999), 36.
3. *Corpus Hermeticum,* Book XII:1, *The Way of Hermes,* 58.
4. *Corpus Hermeticum,* Book XI:4, *The Way of Hermes,* 53.
5. E. J. Holmyard, *Alchemy* (New York: Dover, 1990), 81.
6. See B. J. T. Dobbs, "Newton's *Commentary* on the *Emerald Tablet* of Hermes Trismegistus: Its Scientific and Theological Significance," in Ingrid Merkel and Allen G. Debus, eds., *Hermeticism and the Renaissance: Intellectual History & the Occult in Early Modern Europe* (London and Toronto: Associated University Presses, 1988), 182–91.
7. F. Sherwood Taylor, *The Alchemists: Founders of Modern Chemistry* (London: William Heinemann, 1951), 89–90.
8. Mircea Eliade, *The Forge & the Crucible* (Chicago: University of Chicago Press, 1978), 182–83; H. Stanley Redgrove, *Alchemy, Ancient & Modern* (Wakefield, West Yorkshire, U.K.: EP Publishing, 1973), 13–14.
9. Roger Bacon, *Opera quaedam hactenus inedita,* J. S. Brewer ed., Rolls series, 1859, quoted in Gareth Roberts, *The Mirror of Alchemy* (London: British Library, 1994), 64.
10. J. R. Partington, "The Origins of the Planetary Symbols for the Metals," *Ambix* 1, no. 1 (1937): 61–64.
11. Lily Kolisko, *Workings of the Stars in Earthly Substances* (Stuttgart, Germany: Orient-Occident Verlag, 1928).

12. Ibid.

13. Ibid.; Wilhelm Pelikan, *The Secrets of Metals* (New York: Anthroposophic Press, 1973); Agnes Fyfe, *Moon and Plant* (Arlesheim, Switzerland: Society for Cancer Research, 1975); Nick Kollerstrom, *Astrochemistry: A Study of Metal-Planet Affinities* (London: Emergence Press, 1984).

14. Louise Deacon and Alan Ribot-Smith, *Bellis Perennis: A Proving of a Spagyrically Prepared Sympathetic Medicine* (Tunbridge Wells, England: Helios, 1997); Peter W. Gosch, *Vital Energy Medicine* (Kisslegg, Germany: PEKANA, 2003).

Chapter 2. Paracelsus

1. Carlos Gilly, "Theophrastia Sancta: Paracelsianism as a Religion in Conflict with the Established Churches," in Ole Peter Grell, ed., *Paracelsus: The Man and His Reputation, His Ideas and their Transformation* (Leiden, The Netherlands: E. J. Brill, 1998), 151–86; also at Bibliotheca Philosophia Hermetica, www.ritmanlibrary.nl/c/p/res/art/art_01.html (accessed December 1, 2009).

2. Andrew Cunningham, "Paracelsus Fat and Thin: Thoughts on Reputations and Realities," in Ole Peter Grell, ed., *Paracelsus: The Man and His Reputation, His Ideas and their Transformation* (Leiden, The Netherlands: E. J. Brill, 1998), 53–77.

3. Most notably: Walter Pagel, *Paracelsus: An Introduction to Philosophical Medicine in the Era of the Renaissance,* 2nd ed. (Basel, Switzerland: Karger, 1982); Charles Webster, *From Paracelsus to Newton* (Cambridge: Cambridge University Press, 1982); Andrew Weeks, *Paracelsus: Speculative Theory and the Crisis of the Early Reformation* (New York: SUNY Press, 1997). The most recent is Charles Webster, *Paracelsus: Medicine, Magic and Mission at the End of Time* (New Haven: Yale University Press, 2008).

4. Biographical studies range from the enthusiastic John Hargrave, *The Life and Soul of Paracelsus* (London: Gollancz, 1951), to the theosophical Franz Hartmann, *Life of Paracelsus* (San Diego: Wizards Bookshelf, 1985) and the fuller, more recent assessment of Philip Ball, *The Devil's Doctor: Paracelsus and the World of Renaissance Magic and Science* (London: William Heinemann, 2006).

5. Andrew Weeks, *Paracelsus: Speculative Theory and the Crisis of the Early Reformation,* 10, 84. See also Katharina Biegger, "'De invocatione Beatae Mariae Virginis': Paracelsus und die Marienverehrung," in *Kosmosophie* 6 (1990).

6. Charles Webster, *From Paracelsus to Newton,* 55.

7. National Library of Medicine Exhibition, "Paracelsus and the Medical Revolution of the Renaissance: a 500th Anniversary Celebration by Allen G. Debus," see www.nlm.nih.gov/exhibition/paracelsus/aftermath.html (accessed December 1, 2009).

8. Charles Webster, *From Paracelsus to Newton,* 22. See also Walter Pagel, *Paracelsus: An Introduction to Philosophical Medicine in the Era of the Renaissance,* 211.

9. Philip Ball, *The Devil's Doctor,* 75–79, 94–102. See also endpaper maps.

10. *Liber Paragranum* H.1: 69, in Andrew Weeks, *Paracelsus Theophrastus Bombastus*

von Hohenheim (1493–1541): Essential Theoretical Writings (Leiden, The Netherlands: E. J. Brill, 2008), 303.

11. Many practitioners dipped in and out of academic life: Paracelsus's contemporary, and perhaps the most famous medical practitioner of his generation, Jean Fernel (1497–1558) spent five years out of the university environment in order to pursue private studies. See Linda Deer Richardson, "The Generation of Disease: Occult Causes and Diseases of the Total Substance," in A. Wear, R. K. French, and I. M. Lonie, eds., *The Medical Renaissance of the Sixteenth Century* (Cambridge: Cambridge University Press, 1985), 175–94 (176).

12. G. S. Kirk and J. E. Raven, *The Presocratic Philosophers: A Critical History with a Selection of Texts* (Cambridge: Cambridge University Press, 1960), 328–29.

13. Linda Deer Richardson, "The Generation of Disease," in A. Wear, R. K. French, and I. M. Lonie, eds., *The Medical Renaissance of the Sixteenth Century,* 175–94 (177).

14. Ibid., 180.

15. Ibid.

16. Charles Singer, *A Short History of Medicine* (Oxford: Oxford University Press, 1928), 74.

17. Allen G. Debus, *The French Paracelsians* (Cambridge: Cambridge University Press, 1991), 1.

18. Roger French, "Introduction: The 'Long Fifteenth Century' of Medical History," in Roger French, John Arrizabalaga, Andrew Cunningham, and Luis Garcia-Ballester, eds., *Medicine from the Black Death to the French Disease* (Aldershot, England: Ashgate, 1998), 1–5.

19. Nancy G. Siraisi, "Some Current Trends in the Study of Renaissance Medicine," *Renaissance Quarterly* 37, no. 4 (Winter 1984): 585–600 (586).

20. *De erroribus medicorum secundum fratrem Rogerum Bacon de ordine minorum,* E. T. Withington, trans., "Roger Bacon on the Errors of Physicians," in Charles Singer and Henry E. Sigerist eds., *Essays on the History of Medicine Presented to Karl Sudhoff on the Occasion of His Seventieth Birthday November 26th 1923* (Oxford: Oxford University Press, 1924), 139–57.

21. Michela Pereira, *From the Black Death to the French Disease* (Aldershot, England: Ashgate, 1998), 28–30.

22. Charles Webster, *From Paracelsus to Newton,* 4.

23. Ibid.

24. W. S. C. Copeman, "Medical Education in the Tudor Period," in *Proceedings of the Royal Society of Medicine* 52, no. 8 (1959): 652–60 (657).

25. *Liber Paragranum* H.2:56, in Weeks, *Paracelsus: Essential Theoretical Writings,* 197.

26. George Sarton, *Six Wings: Men of Science in the Renaissance* (London: The Bodley Head, 1958), 105.

27. John Maxson Stillman, "Chemistry and Medicine in the Fifteenth Century," *The Scientific Monthly* 6, no. 2 (1918): 167–75.

28. Walter Pagel, "Medical History at the End of the Nineteenth Century. To Commemorate Julius Pagel (1851–1912) and His Discovery of Medieval Sources," in *Proceedings of the Royal Society of Medicine* 45, no. 5 (1952): 303–6. Michela Pereira also suggests that some forms of alchemy were intended as *scientia experimentalis*, emphasizing Roger Bacon's ideas relating to the perfectibility of matter and of spirit through aequalitas, in her *L'oro dei Filosofi. Saggio sulle idee di un alchimista del Trecento* (Spoleto: n.p., 1992), chap. 2. For Bacon's appreciation of the relationship of medicine and alchemy, see J. S. Brewer, ed., *Opus tertium in Opera Quaedam Hactennus Inedita* (London: Longmans, Green, 1859), vols. 1, 39, and 41.

29. Robert P. Multhauf, "John of Rupescissa and the Origins of Medical Chemistry," *Isis* 45, no. 4 (1954): 359–67 (362).

30. Robert P. Multhauf, *The Origins of Chemistry* (London: Oldbourne, 1966), 179.

31. Robert P. Multhauf, The Relationship between Technology and Natural Philosophy, ca 1250–1650, as Illustrated by the Technology of the Mineral Acids (Ph.D. dissertation, University of California, 1953), 33–92.

32. *Calendar of Patent Rolls,* quoted in Michela Pereira, *"Mater Medicinarum:* English Physicians and the Alchemical Elixir in the Fifteenth Century," in Roger French, et. al., *Medicine from the Black Death to the French Disease,* 26–52 (26).

33. F. Rafail Farag, "Why Europe Responded to the Muslims' Medical Achievements in the Middle Ages," *Arabica* 25, no. 3 (1978): 292–309 (297, 301).

34. Allen G. Debus, *The French Paracelsians,* 50.

35. Bernard D. Haage, "Alchemy II: Antiquity–12th Century," in Wouter J. Hanegraaff, Antoine Faivre, Roelof van den Broek, and Jean-Pierre Brach, eds., *Dictionary of Gnosis and Western Esotericism* (Leiden, The Netherlands: E. J. Brill, 2005), I, 16–34 (20).

36. W. S. C. Copeman, "Medical Education in the Tudor Period," *Proceedings of the Royal Society of Medicine* 52, no. 8 (1959): 652–80 (653).

37. Charles Webster, "Alchemical and Paracelsian Medicine," in Charles Webster, ed., *Health, Medicine and Mortality in the Sixteenth Century* (Cambridge: Cambridge University Press, 1979), 302.

38. Faye Marie Getz, "To Prolong Life and Promote Health: Baconian Alchemy and Pharmacy in the English Learned Tradition," in Sheila Campbell, Bert Hall, David Klausner, eds., *Health, Disease and Healing in Medieval Culture* (Basingstoke, England: Macmillan, 1992), 141–51.

39. Roger French, et al., *Medicine from the Black Death to the French Disease,* 27.

40. Haage, "Alchemy II," 21. See also Michela Pereira, *Medicine from the Black Death to the French Disease,* 28.

41. Antonio Clericuzio, "Chemical Medicine and Paracelsianism in Italy 1550–1650," in Margaret Pelling and Scott Mandelbrote, eds., *The Practice of Reform in Health, Medicine and Science, 1500–2000: Essays for Charles Webster* (Aldershot, England: Ashgate, 2005), 59–80.

Chapter 3. Paracelsian Philosophy
and Spagyric Alchemy

1. Hans Fischer "Die kosmologische Anthropologie des Paracelsus als Grundlage seiner Medizin," *Verh. Naturforsch. Ges. Basel* 52 (1941): 189ff; cit. Walter Pagel, *Paracelsus,* 348.

2. Jolande Jacobi, *Paracelsus: Selected Writings* (Princeton, N.J.: Princeton University Press, 1958), 68.

3. Allen G. Debus, *The Chemical Philosophy* (Mineola, N.Y.: Dover, 1977), 56–57.

4. *Liber Paragranum* H.2:40, in Weeks, *Paracelsus: Essential Theoretical Writings,* 159.

5. Ibid., H.2:29, 129.

6. Ibid., H.2:24, 113–15.

7. Daniel Sennert, *The Weapon-Salve Maladie* (London: n.p., 1637), 4f.

8. James McEvoy, *The Philosophy of Robert Grosseteste* (Oxford: Oxford University Press, 1982), 180–88.

9. *Liber Paragranum* H.2:23, in Weeks, *Paracelsus: Essential Theoretical Writings,* 113.

10. D. P. Walker, "The Astral Body in Renaissance Medicine," *Journal of the Warburg and Courtauld Institutes* 21, no. 1–2 (1968): 119–33 (122).

11. *Liber Azoth* (1591), in Allen G. Debus, *Chemical Philosophy,* 87.

12. *Liber Paragranum,* H.2:44, in Weeks, *Paracelsus: Essential Theoretical Writings,* 167–69.

13. *Volumen Medicinae Paramirum* (ca. 1520), in Nicholas Goodrick-Clarke, *Paracelsus: Essential Readings* (Berkeley, Calif.: North Atlantic, 1999), 45.

14. Allen G. Debus, *Chemical Philosophy,* 53, 88.

15. Nicholas Goodrick-Clarke, *Paracelsus: Essential Readings,* 112–13.

16. Ibid., 26–27.

17. Ibid., 24–33.

18. Paracelsus, *Liber de Imaginibus,* in *The Prophecies of Paracelsus,* J. K., trans. (New York: Weiser, 1974), 35.

19. *Liber Paragranum* H.2:18, in Weeks, *Paracelsus: Essential Theoretical Writings,* 97–99.

20. Ibid., H.2:66, 220–21.

21. Sir Thomas Browne, *Pseudoxia epidemica,* in *Works* 2, 261.

22. Jan Baptista van Helmont, *Oriatrike or Physick Redefined,* John Chandler, trans. (London: n.p., 1664), V, 35.

23. Emmanuel Swedenborg, *Economy of the Animal Kingdom* I. § 253; cit. Martin Lamm, *Emanuel Swedenborg: The Development of His Thought* (West Chester, Pa.: Swedenborg Foundation, 2000), 69.

24. Walter Pagel, *Paracelsus,* 349.

25. Paracelsus, *Astronomia* H.2:26, in Weeks, *Paracelsus: Essential Theoretical Writings,* 197.

26. Walter Pagel, "Jung's Views on Alchemy," *Isis* 39, no. 1–2 (May 1948): 44–48.

27. Jacobi, *Paracelsus,* 21.

28. Sir Isaac Newton, MS of *Latin Opticks* (1706), 3970, f.619.

29. Richard Gerber, *Vibrational Medicine* (Sante Fe: Bear & Company, 1988), 40.

Chapter 4. The Vital Force:
Samuel Hahnemann and Homeopathy

1. Clare Goodrick-Clarke, "Rationalist, Empiricist, or *Naturphilosoph*? Samuel Hahnemann and his Legacy," *Politica Hermetica* 18 (2004): 26–45.

2. Samuel Hahnemann, *Organon of Medicine,* R. E. Dudgeon and William Boericke, trans. (New Delhi: B. Jain, 1995), §6, p. 32.

3. Samuel Hahnemann, "Observations on the Three Current Methods of Treatment" (1809), in *Lesser Writing,* R. E. Dudgeon, ed., trans. (New Delhi: B. Jain, 1995), 533.

4. Samuel Hahnemann, *The Organon of the Medical Art,* Stephen Decker, trans., Wenda Brewster O'Reilly, ed. (Palo Alto, Calif.: Birdcage Books, 1996), 9.

5. Ibid., 66–69.

6. James Tyler Kent, *Lectures on Homeopathic Philosophy* (New Delhi: B. Jain, 1995), 73, 90.

7. Ralph Twentyman, *The Science and Art of Healing* (Edinburgh: Floris Books, 1989), 18.

8. James Tyler Kent, *Lectures on Homeopathic Philosophy,* 86.

9. Ibid., 94.

10. Francis Treuherz, "Hecla Lava, or the Influence of Swedenborg on Homeopathy," *The Homeopath* 4, no. 2 (1983): 35–50 (50).

11. James Tyler Kent, *Lectures on Homeopathic Philosophy,* 24.

12. Ernst Benz, *Emanuel Swedenborg: Visionary Seer in the Age of Reason,* Nicholas Goodrick-Clarke, trans. (West Chester, Pa.: Swedenborg Foundation, 2002), 131.

13. James Tyler Kent, *Lectures on Homeopathic Philosophy,* 21.

14. Ibid., 73.

15. Samuel Hahnemann, *The Organon of the Medical Art,* Stephen Decker, trans., Wenda Brewster O'Reilly, ed. (Palo Alto, Calif.: Birdcage Books, 1996), 58.

16. Edzard Ernst, *Trick or Treatment: Alternative Medicine on Trial* (London: Bantam, 2008), 104.

17. James Tyler Kent, *Lectures on Homeopathic Philosophy,* 77.

18. Ibid., 70.

19. Ibid., 70–74.

20. Richard Gerber, *Vibrational Medicine* (Santa Fe: Bear and Co., 1988), 41.

21. Stuart Close, *The Genius of Homeopathy* (New Delhi: B. Jain, 1996), 77

22. Ibid., 76.

23. Ibid., 78–79.

24. Samuel Hahnemann, "The Lesser Writings," in Harris Coulter, *The Divided Legacy,* 4 vols. (Berkeley, Calif.: North Atlantic, 1975–1994), II, 389.

25. Richard Grossinger, *Homeopathy: An Introduction for Sceptics and Beginners* (Berkeley: North Atlantic Books, 1993), 58.

26. Thorwald Dethlefsen and Rüdiger Dahlke, *The Healing Power of Illness* (Shaftesbury, England: Element, 1990), 88.

27. Ibid., 58.

28. Richard Grossinger, *Homeopathy: An Introduction for Sceptics and Beginners,* 55.

29. Stuart Close, *The Genius of Homeopathy,* 75

30. Edward Bach, letter written to colleagues in 1935, in Julian Barnard, ed., *Collected Writings of Edward Bach* (Hereford, England: Flower Remedy Programme, 1987), 23.

Chapter 5. Neo-Paracelsian Spagyrics

1. Christopher McIntosh, *The Rose Cross and the Age of Reason* (Leiden, The Netherlands: E. J. Brill, 1992).

2. Clare Goodrick-Clarke, "Rationalist, Empiricist, or *Naturphilosoph?* Samuel Hahnemann and His Legacy," 26–45.

3. A. A. Ramseyer, ed., *Rademacher's Universal and Organ Remedies* (New Delhi: B. Jain, 1999), 100.

4. H. L. Chitkara, ed., *The Best of Burnett,* comp. H. L. Chitkara (New Delhi: B. Jain, 1995), viii.

5. Ibid., xi.

6. Ibid., 96.

7. Ibid.

8. Ibid.

9. Ibid., 47.

10. Ibid., 94.

11. Ibid., 111.

12. Ibid., 47.

13. This was the opinion of his friend and biographer, Dr. J. H. Clarke cit. ibid., vi.

14. For details of Zimpel's biography, see Axel Helmstädter, *Spagyrische Arzneimittel,* 83–99.

15. Ibid., 107.

16. Libavius, *Alchemie* (1597), reprinted Weinheim, 1964.

17. Manfred M. Junius, *Spagyrics: The Alchemical Preparation of Medical Essences, Tinctures, and Elixirs* (Rochester, Vt.: Healing Arts Press, 2007).

18. Peter W. Gosch, *Vital Energy Medicine* (Kissleg, Germany: PEKANA, 2003), 18–19.

19. Ibid., 79.

20. Maximilian Bircher-Benner, *Vom Werden des Neuen Artztes* (Dresden: Wilhelm Heyne Verlag, 1938), 122; cit. Gosch, *Vital Energy Medicine,* 79.

Chapter 6. Making Spagyric Essences

1. Manfred M. Junius, *Spagyrics: The Alchemical Preparation of Medicinal Essences, Tinctures and Elixirs* (Rochester, Vt.: Healing Arts Press, 2007), 24.
2. Franz Hartmann, *The Life of Paracelsus* (San Diego: Wizard's Bookshelf, 1985), 209–10.

Chapter 7. Plant Profiles and Therapeutics

1. A. A. Ramseyer, *Rademacher's Universal and Organ Remedies* (New Delhi: B. Jain, 1999), 22.
2. John Gerard, *Great Herbal* (London: Norton, 1597).
3. Wighard Strehlow, *Hildegard of Bingen's Spiritual Remedies* (Rochester Vt.: Healing Arts Press, 2002), 76.
4. Nicolas Culpeper, *The English Physitian* (London: Peter Cole, 1652), 51.
5. Frans Vermeulen, *Concordant Materia Medica* (Haarlem, The Netherlands: Emryss Publishers, 2000), 704.
6. Paracelsus, in Franz Hartmann, *The Life of Paracelsus* (San Diego: Wizards Bookshelf, 1985), 140–41.
7. Nicholas Culpeper, *Complete Herbal and English Physician* (London: 1653), 36.
8. John Gerard, *Great Herbal* (London: Norton, 1597).
9. See Frank Shallenberger, *The Type 2 Diabetes Breakthrough* (Laguna Beach, Calif.: Basic Health Publications, 2006).
10. Culpeper, *Complete Herbal and English Physician,* 165.

Bibliography

Energy Medicine

Dethlefsen, Thorwald, and Rüdiger Dahlke. *The Healing Power of Illness: The Meaning of Symptoms and How to Interpret Them.* Shaftesbury, England: Element, 1990.

Gerber, Richard. *Vibrational Medicine.* Sante Fe: Bear and Co., 1988.

Flower Essences and Herbs

Bach, Edward. *Collected Writings.* Hereford, England: Flower Remedy Programme, 1987.

Barnard, Julian, and Martine Barnard. *Healing Herbs of Edward Bach.* Hereford, England: Bach Educational Programme, 1988.

Bartram, Thomas. *Encyclopedia of Herbal Medicine.* London: Robinson, 1995.

Bown, Deni. *The Royal Horticultural Society Encyclopedia of Herbs and Their Uses.* London: Dorling Kindersley, 1995.

British Herbal Medicine Association. *British Herbal Phamocopoeia,* 2 vols. London: British Herbal Medicine Association, 1976.

Compton Burnett, James. *The Best of Burnett.* Edited by H. L. Chitkara. New Delhi: B. Jain, 1995.

———. *Diseases of the Spleen.* New Delhi: B. Jain, 2003.

Culpeper, Nicholas. *Complete Herbal.* Birmingham: Imperial Chemical (Pharmaceuticals), Ltd., 1953.

Frawley, David, and Vasant Lad. *Yoga of Herbs: An Ayurvedic Guide to Herbal Medicine.* Twin Lakes, Wis.: Lotus Press, 1992.

Grieve, M. *A Modern Herbal,* 2 vols. Toronto: Jonathan Cape, 1931.

Lewis, Walter H., and Memory P. F. Elvin-Lewis. *Medical Botany: Plants Affecting Man's Health.* New York: John Wiley and Sons, 1977.

Murphy, Robin. *Lotus Materia Medica: Homeopathic and Spagyric Medicines.* Pagosa Springs, Colo.: Lotus Star Academy, 1995.

Ramseyer, A. A. *Rademacher's Universal and Organ Remedies.* New Delhi: B. Jain, 1999.

Scholten, Jan. *Minerals in Plants,* 2 vols. Utrecht: Stichting Alannissos, 2002.

Smith, Ed. *Therapeutic Herb Manual.* Williams, Ore.: Ed Smith, 1999.

Strehlow, Wighard, and Gottfried Hertzka. *Hildegard of Bingen's Medicine.* Santa Fe: Bear and Co., 1988.

Stuart, Malcolm, ed. *Encyclopedia of Herbs & Herbalism.* London: Orbis, 1979.

Vermeulen, Franz. *Concordant Materia Medica.* Haarlem, the Netherlands: Emryss Publishers, 2000.

————. *Prisma: The Arcana of Meteria Medica Illuminated.* Haarlem, the Netherlands: Emryss Publishers, 2002.

————. *Synoptic Materia Medica 2.* Haarlem, the Netherlands: Merlijn Publishers, 1996.

Wood, Matthew. *Seven Herbs: Plants as Teachers.* Berkeley, Calif.: North Atlantic, 1987.

————. *The Book of Herbal Wisdom: Using Plants as Medicines.* Berkeley, Calif.: North Atlantic, 1997.

Woodward, Marcus, ed. *Gerard's Herbal.* London: Studio Editions, 1994.

Worwood, Valerie Ann. *The Fragrant Heavens: The Spiritual Dimension of Fragrance and Aromatherapy.* New York: Doubleday, 1999.

Hahnemann and Homeopathy

Boericke, William. *Materia Medica.* New Delhi: B. Jain, 1996.

Close, Stuart. *The Genius of Homeopathy.* New Delhi: B. Jain, 1996.

Coulter, Harris. *The Divided Legacy: A History of the Schism in Medical Thought,* 4 vols. Berkeley, Calif.: North Atlantic, 1975–1994.

————. *Homeopathic Science and Modern Medicine: The Physics of Healing with Microdoses.* Berkeley, Calif.: North Atlantic, 1981.

Goodrick-Clarke, Clare. "Rationalist, Empiricist, or *Naturphilosoph*?: Samuel Hahnemann and His Legacy." In *Politica Hermetica* 18 (2004): 26–45.

Grossinger, Richard. *Homeopathy: An Introduction for Sceptics and Beginners.* Berkeley, Calif.: North Atlantic Books, 1993.

Haehl, Richard. *Samuel Hahnemann: His Life and Work,* 2 vols. New Delhi: B. Jain, 2003.

Hahnemann, Samuel. *The Organon of the Medical Art.* Edited by Wenda Brewster O'Reilly. Translated by Stephen Decker. Palo Alto, Calif.: Birdcage Books, 1996.

————. *Lesser Writings.* Translated by R. E. Dudgeon. New Delhi: B. Jain, 1995.

Kent, James Tyler. *Lectures on Homeopathic Philosophy.* New Delhi: B. Jain, 1995.

Lessell, Colin B. *A New Physics of Homeopathy.* Leigh-on-Sea, England: Alliance of Registered Homeopaths, 2002.

Roberts, H. A. *The Principles and Art of Cure by Homeopathy.* New Delhi: B. Jain, 1996.

Schiff, Michel. *The Memory of Water: Homeopathy and the Battle of Ideas in the New Science*. London: Thorsons, 1995.

Whitmont, Edward C. *Psyche and Substance: Essays on Homeopathy in the Light of Jungian Psychology*. Berkeley, Calif.: North Atlantic Books, 1980.

Paracelsus

Ball, Philip. *The Devil's Doctor: Paracelsus and the World of Renaissance Magic & Science*. London: William Heinemann, 2006.

Coudert, Allison. "Alchemy IV: 15th–18th Century." In *Dictionary of Gnosis & Western Esotericism*, 2 vols. Edited by Wouter Hanegraaff, et al. Leiden, the Netherlands: E. J. Brill, 2005.

Debus, Allen G. *The English Paracelsians*. New York: Franklin Watts, 1966.

———. "Renaissance Chemistry and the Work of Robert Fludd." *Ambix* 14, no. 1 (1967): 42–59.

———. *The Chemical Philosophy: Paracelsian Science and Medicine in the Sixteenth and Seventeenth Centuries*. Mineoloa, N.Y.: Dover Publications, 2002. First published in 2 vols. in 1977.

Goodrick-Clarke, Nicholas. *Paracelsus: Essential Readings*. Berkeley, Calif.: North Atlantic Press, 1999.

Hargrave, John. *The Life and Soul of Paracelsus*. London: Victor Gollancz, 1951.

Jacobi, Jolande. *Paracelsus: Selected Writings*. Princeton, N.J.: Princeton University Press, 1973.

Pagel, Walter. *Paracelsus: An Introduction to Philosophical Medicine in the Era of the Renaissance*, 2nd ed. Basel, Switzerland: Karger, 1982.

———. "The Prime Matter of Paracelsus." *Ambix* 9, no. 3 (1961): 117–35.

———. "Paracelsus and the Neoplatonic and Gnostic Tradition." *Ambix* 8, no. 3 (1960): 125–66.

Rattansi, Piyo, and Antonio Clericuzio, eds. *Alchemy and Chemistry in the 16th and 17th centuries*. Dordrecht, the Netherlands: Kluwer Academic Publishers, 1994.

Schipperges, Heinrich. "Paracelsus and His Followers." In Faivre, Antoine, and Jacob Needleman, eds. *Modern Esoteric Spirituality*. London: SCM Press, 1993, 154–85.

Sherlock, T. P. "The Chemical Work of Paracelsus." *Ambix* 3, no. 1–2 (1948): 33–63.

Shumaker, Wayne. *The Occult Sciences in the Renaissance: A Study in Intellectual Patterns*. Berkeley, Calif.: University of California Press, 1972.

Thorndike, Lynn. "Alchemy During the First Half of the Sixteenth Century." *Ambix* 2, no. 1 (1938): 26–37.

Voss, Karen-Claire. "Spiritual Alchemy: Interpreting Representative Texts and Images." In Van den Broek, Roelof, and Wouter J. Hanegraaff, eds. *Gnosis and Hermeticism from Antiquity to Modern Times*. Albany, N.Y.: SUNY Press, 1998, 147–81.

Weeks, Andrew. *Paracelsus: Speculative Theory & the Crisis of the Early Reformation*. Albany, N.Y.: SUNY Press, 1997.

———. *Paracelsus (Theophrastus Bombastus von Hohenheim, 1493–1541): Essential Theoretical Writings.* Leiden, the Netherlands: E. J. Brill, 2008.

Practical Alchemy and Neo-Paracelsian Spagyrics

Albertus, Frater. *The Alchemist's Handbook.* York Beach, Maine: Samuel Weiser, 1998.

———. *Praxis Spagyrica Philosophica.* York Beach, Maine: Samuel Weiser, 1974.

Bernus, Alexander von. *Alchymie und Heilkunst.* Privately printed, 1936; reprinted by Dornach: Rudolf Geering Verlag, 1994.

Cotnoir, Brian. *Alchemy.* York Beach, Maine: Samuel Weiser, 2006.

Danciger, Elizabeth. *Homeopathy from Alchemy to Medicine.* Rochester, Vt.: Healing Arts Press, 1988.

Fritschi, Hans-Joseph. *Spagyrik: Lehr- und Arbeitsbuch* [*Spagyrics: A Workbook*]. Ulm, Germany: Gustav Fischer Verlag, 1997.

Gebelein, Helmut. *Alchemie.* Munich: Heinrich Hugendubel Verlag, 1991.

Gosch, Peter W. *Vital Energy Medicine.* Kisslegg, Germany: PEKANA, 2003.

Helmstädter, Axel. *Spagyrische Arzneimittel: Pharmazie und Alchemie der Neuzeit* [Spagyric Healing: Pharmacy and Alchemy in Modernity]. Stuttgart: Wissenschaftliche Verlagsgesellschaft, 1990.

Junius, Manfred M. *Spagyrics: The Alchemical Preparation of Medicinal Essences, Tinctures and Elixirs.* Rochester, Vt.: Healing Arts Press, 2007.

Leibbrand, Werner. *Romantische Medizin* [Romantic Medicine]. Hamburg: H. Goverts, 1937.

Richter, Herta, and Michael Schünemann. *Spagirisch heilen: Die JSO-Komplex-Heilweise* [Spagyric Healing: The ISO-Complex Healing Method]. Munich: Foitzick Verlag, 2000.

Rippe, Olaf, et al. *Paracelsusmedizin: Altes Wissen in der Heilkunst von heute* [Paracelsian Medicine: Ancient Knowledge in the Healing Arts of Today]. Aarau, Germany: AT Verlag, 2001.

Surya, G. W. *Die Spagyriker: Paracelsus—Rademacher—Zimpel* [The Spagyric Practitioners: Paracelsus, Rademacher, and Zimpel]. Berlin-Pankow: Linser-Verlag, 1923.

Wood, Matthew. *The Magical Staff: The Vitalist Tradition in Western Medicine.* Berkeley, Calif.: North Atlantic Books, 1992.

Resources

Alchemy

The Alchemy website:
www.levity.com/alchemy

The Alchemy Museum at Kutna Hora:
www.alchemy.cz/museum.html

Spagyric Essences

Australerba Herbal Products and Spagyric laboratories:
www.australerba.com.au/

Online store for spagyric remedies and resources in the USA:
www.spagyrium.com

Homeopathic and Spagyric Medications

Lemasor Gmbh
Bergstrasse 19
D-66346 Püttlingen Germany
www.lemasor.com

Phylak-Sachsen
PHYLAK Sachsen (Schweiz) Gmbh
Gotthelfstrasse 34
3432 Lütwelflüh Switzerland
Phone: + 41-34-4616-288
www.phylak@bluewin.ch
PHYLAK Germany: www.phylak.com
www.spagyricmedicine.com

Soluna Spagyrics
Laboratorium SOLUNA Heilmittel Gmbh
Artur-Proellerstrasse 9
96609 Donauwörth Germany
www.soluna.com

Soluna in the United States:
USA Innovative Medicine Inc.
303 Fifth Avenue, Suite 1906
New York, NY 10016
Phone: 800-605-1798
www.solunalabs.com

PEKANA Homeopathic-Spagryic Medications
BioResource Inc.
321 Blodgett Street, Suite B
Cotati, CA 94931
Phone: 800-203-3775
www.bioresource.com

Herbs

In Harmony Herbs & Spices
P.O. Box 7555
San Diego, CA 92167
Phone: 619-223-8051
www.inharmonyherbs.com

Planetary Herbal Products
P.O. Box 779
Brookdale, CA 95007
Phone: 408-338-1305
www.planetaryherbs.com

History of Homeopathy and Biographies of Homeopaths

http://homeopathy.wildfalcon.com

Index

Index of Plants—Latin Names

Achillea millefolium (yarrow), 108–11, 122
Arnica, 113
Bellis perennis (daisy), 113
Calendula officinalis (calendula), 111–15, 140
Carduus marianus (St. Mary's Thistle), 115–18
Ceanothus americanus (ceanothus), 118–21
Chamomilla (chamomile), 121–25
Chelidonium majus, 116
Crataegus oxyacanthoides (hawthorn), 125–28
Digitalis (foxglove), 8, 126
Equisetum arvense (horsetail), 128–31
Euphrasia (eyebright), 28, 83
Foeniculum vulgare (fennel), 131–34
Galium asparine (cleavers), 98, 101, 134–37
Hypericum perforatum (St. John's wort), 10, 23, 137–40, 144
Iris Versicolor (iris), 141–44
Matricaria recutita. See Chamomilla
Melissa officinalis (lemon balm), 144–47
Rosmarinus officinalis (rosemary), 25, 107, 134, 147–50
Salvia officinalis (sage), 5, 150–54, 160
Sambucus nigra (elderflower), 153–56, 164
Taraxacum officinale (dandelion), 9, 10, 137, 157–60
Urtica dioica (stinging nettle) 10, 11, 137, 160–64

Index of Plants—Common Names

agrimony, 10
calendula, 107, 111–15, 140
ceanothus, 118–21
chamomile, 121–25
chickweed, 11
cleavers, 98, 101, 134–37
clover, 10
dandelion, 9, 10, 137, 157–60
elderflower, 153–56, 164
eyebright, 28, 83
fennel, 131–34
goldenrod, 10
hawthorn, 11, 125–28, 147, 155
horsetail, 128–31
iris, 141–44
lemon balm, 144
mint, 5
mullein, 10
nettle, 10, 11, 137, 160–64
plantain, 10, 11
poppies, 10
rosemary, 25, 107, 134, 147–50
sage, 5, 150–54, 160
St. John's wort, 10, 23, 137–40, 144
St. Mary's thistle, 115–17
sunflower, 10
teasle, 10
wild orchid, 10
wild rose, 12
yarrow, 108–11, 156, 164

General Index

Achilles, 72, 109
action at a distance, 49–50
acupuncture, 2, 74
Ader, Robert, 72
Aerial Niter, 53–54
Albertus Magnus, 13, 23
Alchemy, origins of, 15, 17
alcohol, 3, 28, 29, 30, 44, 67, 88, 89, 93, 97, 99, 102, 103, 106, 107, 117, 129, 139, 161, 162

Alexandria, 14, 15, 17, 35, 38, 39
allopathy (healing by contraries), 2, 41, 73
Ancient & Mystical Order of the Rose
    Crucis (AMORC), 90
Andreä, Johannes Valentin, 79–81
Anima mundi, 57
Apollonius of Tyana, 20–21
Arcana, 56, 57
Archeus, 43, 47, 56, 57, 58, 70
Arnau de Vilanova, 23, 42, 45, 46
Aristotle, 13, 24, 35, 39, 50
Asclepius, 57
astral body, 47, 51–54, 56
astro-chemistry, 26
astrology, 13, 15, 20, 24, 34, 35, 43, 44, 46,
    53, 54, 55, 90, 99, 150
Avicenna, 13, 35, 37, 38, 45–46, 48, 56, 145

Babylonia, 15, 16, 24
Bach, Edward, 12
Bacon, Roger, 13, 23, 42, 45, 46
Bernus, Alexander von, 92
Beyersdorff, Peter, 93
Black Death (1348), 41. *See also* plague
Boehme, Jacob, 62, 65, 66, 79, 81, 87, 92
Bolos of Mendes. *See* Democritus
Bönschen, Thomas, 93
Boyle, Sir Robert, 13, 39, 78
Brahe, Tycho, 44, 79
Browne, Sir Thomas, 57
Brynschwyg, Hieronymous, 44, 45
Byzantium, 17, 39

calcination, 12, 19, 29, 30, 31, 88, 93, 98, 99,
    103, 104, 105
Calvin, Jean, 33
capillary dynamolysis, 26–27
Caput mortuum (death's head), 12, 29, 104
Celsus, 24, 35, 37
Champier, Symphorien, 35
chemical marriage, 9, 17, 22, 30
Christ, 19, 30, 37, 154
Christianity, 13, 14, 15, 17, 30, 33, 34, 45, 51
Circulatum minus, 91
Cochrane Institute, 139
Compton Burnett, James, 84, 85, 119, 119

Constantinus Africanus, 39, 44
Copernicus, 34, 35, 44
Corpus Hermeticum, 15–20, 25, 27
correspondences, 15, 28, 50, 55, 83
Cosimo de' Medici, 17, 35
crystal therapy, 2
Culpeper, Nicholas, 109, 111, 115, 116, 127,
    131, 133, 146, 147, 148, 150, 163

Democritus (Pseudo-Democritus a.k.a.
    Bolos of Mendes), 16, 18
Dioscorides, 35, 115, 116, 126
dissolution, 19, 45, 92
distillation, 12, 28–31, 44–45, 49, 88, 93,
    98, 99, 104, 105, 106, 107, 110, 154
Doctrine of Signatures, 27, 28, 54, 83, 109,
    138, 157
Dorn, Gerard, 30
dynamic forces in Nature, 12, 29, 52, 54, 58

electrohomeopathy, 87, 89
elixir, 16, 45, 46, 80, 91, 145
Emerald Tablet, 15, 20, 21
Empedocles, 39, 40
Erasmus, Desiderius, 33, 37
esoteric alchemy, 23

fermentation, 29, 30, 89, 93
Fernel, Jean, 44, 52
Ficino, Marsilio, 18, 35
filtration, 12, 29, 31, 96, 103
five element theory, 159
Flower Remedies, 12, 31, 77, 97
Fludd, Robert, 50, 80
four element theory, 24, 39, 40, 48, 49, 51
Four Humors, 39, 40–43, 148
four pillars of medicine, 43
Freemasonry, 61, 62
Froben, 37
Fyfe, Agnes, 27

Galen, 34, 35–41, 56, 135, 145
Geber (Latin Geber), 45
Georgiewitz-Weitzer, Demeter (G. W.
    Surya), 92
Gerard of Cremona, 39

Gerard, John, 117, 132, 135, 151, 162
Gerber, Richard, 59, 71
Glückselig, Conrad Johann, 92
Gnosticism, 14, 15, 17, 18, 45
God, 18, 27, 28, 43
Goethe, 80, 81, 82, 92
gold, 16, 17, 22, 23, 25, 29
  of higher consciousness, 22
Great Work, 16, 50
Greek myths, 141
Greek philosophy, 15, 18
Grosseteste, Robert, 13, 50
Guinther of Andernach, 41

Hahnemann, Samuel, 60–77, 80, 82, 83, 87, 89
  bacteria as scavengers of disease, 64
  early life, 60
  Freemasonry, 61
  motto, 60
  medical studies, 61
  new medical system, 61–62, 64
  translator, 61
herbalism, 2, 9, 29, 31, 74
Henry VII, King of England, 41
Henry VIII, King of England, 41
Hermes, 14, 15, 20, 21, 22, 27, 29, 30. 141
Hermetic philosophy, 13–21, 29, 47, 58, 59, 79, 80, 81, 89, 93, 153
Hermetic project, 19, 20, 21
Hildegard of Bingen, 33, 36, 132, 133
Hippocrates, 4, 35, 38, 41, 43, 53, 69
homeopathy, 2, 4, 29, 31, 32, 38. 40, 41, 57, 60–68, 70, 73–75, 78, 81, 84–89, 93, 97, 98, 105, 119, 120, 160, 162
homeopathic
  dilution, 41, 66–68, 98, 105
  potency, 62, 64, 66, 67–68, 72, 75, 97, 105, 120
  principles, 31, 68, 69,
  provings, 6, 69
  spagyrics, 31, 37, 93
Holmyard, E. J., 30
Hufeland, Christoph, 61, 82
Hugo of Santalla, 21
Hunayn ibn Ishaq, 39

iatrochemistry, 32, 78, 79, 83, 84
iatrogenic disease, 2, 75
imagination, 54, 44, 58
immateriality of disease, 52, 60, 62, 64, 65, 70, 72, 73, 75, 77

Jabir ibn Hayyan, 20
Jewish Mysticism, 13, 14, 17, 43. 161
John of Rupescissa, 23
Jung, Carl Gustav, 31
Junius, Manfred, 91, 96

Kabbalah, 14
Kent, James Tyler, 64–69, 71, 73
Kepler, Johannes, 44, 79
Khunrath, Heinrich, 30
Kirlian photography, 31
Kolisko, Lily, 26, 27
Krauss, Theodor, 89

Lemasor, 93
Libavius, Andreas, 91
Light of Nature, 30. 36, 55, 77
Llull, Ramon, 23, 46
Luther, Martin, 33, 34, 79

macrocosm-microcosm, 20, 28, 29, 36, 40, 47, 48, 49, 50, 51, 52, 54, 55, 58, 59
Magia naturalis, 45
magic, 15, 45, 46, 48, 50, 51, 54, 70, 79, 81
Magistery, 3, 29, 31
Mattei, Count Cesare, 89, 116
Mead, G. R. S., 93
medicinal alchemy, 12, 46, 47
mercury (metal), 24, 25, 28, 29, 30, 45, 47, 55, 56, 61, 78, 93, 97, 103, 125, 139
Mercury (planet), 24, 121, 124, 125, 131, 133, 135, 147, 151, 153, 156
Mesmer, Franz Anton, 69, 81
metal salts, 26
mineral acids, 45
Mondeville, Henri de, 40
Moon, phases of, 100
Morienus, 50
Mysterium magnum, 48

Naidu, George, 93
Naturphilosophie (German Romantic
    Natural Science), 62, 64, 78, 80, 82,
    88
Neoplatonism, 14, 15, 18, 45, 48, 51, 58,
    90, 81
Newton, Sir Isaac, 13, 21, 59
Nous, 18, 19, 20, 27
North American Indians, 109, 118, 141,
    142, 151

Paracelsus, 3, 13, 28–31, 32–59, 60, 66, 68,
    79, 73, 77–90. 92, 93 145
    Basle, 37
    death in Salzburg, 37
    early life, 33
    Ens of disease, 43
    four pillars of medicine, 43
    later influence, 78–94
    Light of Nature, 77
    medicine in his time, 35–36, 38
    Melissa spagyric essence, 106
    motto, 9
    peregrination, 36
    prayer, 102
    theory of disease, 42–44
    small doses of medicine, 79
    use of *Hypericum,* 136
Paracelsus College, 90
Paracelsus Research Society, 90
Pekana, 93
Periodic Table, 28
Philosophy of Nature, 16, 54
Phönix, 92
phytotherapeutics, 3, 8, 9, 12, 31, 88, 89, 97
Pietism, 60, 62, 64, 65, 80, 88
Pincaldi, Augusto, 91
placebo, 57, 69, 139, 162
Plague, 41, 43. 45. *See also* Black Death
planets, 15, 24, 26, 28, 121, 125, 128, 131,
    134, 145, 152
planetary metals, 24, 25, 26–27, 28
Prima material, 19, 42, 58
Plato, 17, 18, 24, 35, 47, 48
Platonic Academy, 35
Pliny, 116, 135, 145, 162

polarity, 75, 76, 81
Proeller family, 92
Provers' Union, 69
Ptolemy, 24
putrefaction, 19

Quest Society, 93

Rademacher, Gottfried, 82–87, 116, 119
reflexology, 2
Reformation, 33, 34
Renaissance, 29, 34, 39, 42, 51, 116
Rhazes, 23, 45
Richert, Karl, 92
Riedel, Albert Richard (Frater Albertus), 90
Rosicrucian movement, 32, 61, 80, 81, 90,
    92
Royal London Homoeopathic Hospital, 86

Saint Mary the Virgin, 33, 34, 112, 115, 124
Saint Paul, 14, 19
salts, 30, 31, 48, 55, 91, 97, 104
    metallic salts 26
    mineral salts 26
    salt water 31
    soluble salts (electrolytes) 3, 28, 29, 88,
        98
separation, 42, 48
solution, 26, 27, 42, 85, 88, 164
sublimation, 52, 104
sulphur, 17, 22
Sun in Aries, 150
Surya. *See* Georgiewitz-Weitzer
Scot, Michael, 23, 45
similars, 4, 38, 51, 68, 87
Similimum, 47, 60
Solaria, 92
Soluna, 92
Spiritus mundi, 51
Stahl, Georg Ernst, 69, 116, 117
Starkey, George, 57, 78
Steiner, Rudolf, 81, 92
Swedenborg, Emanuel, 57, 58, 64, 65, 66,
    68
Swedenborgianism, 64, 65, 66, 87
symbols, 15, 19, 24, 28, 29

Theophrastia sancta, 32
Theosophy, 61, 79, 87, 93
Theosophical Society, 81
Thoth, 14
tinctures, 16, 18, 25, 28, 29, 31, 57, 120, 138, 161
transmutation, 17, 20, 22, 23, 58, 54, 57, 130
Traditional Chinese Medicine, 2, 74, 119, 159
Tria prima, 28, 29, 30, 31, 46, 47, 55, 56, 78, 91
Trithemius, Johann, 36

universities
  Bologna, 40, 42, 45
  Cambridge, 46
  Erlangen, 61
  Ferrara, 40
  Montpellier, 40, 42, 45, 46
  Oxford, 40, 46
  Padua, 49, 41
  Paris, 49
Unmanifest, 19, 27
Urbigerus, Baron, 91

Van Helmont, Jan Baptista, 39, 57, 58, 66, 78, 79
Vesalius, 34, 35, 41
Vienna Medical School, 35, 61, 69, 85
Vis formatrix, 58, 71
Vis plastica, 58
vital force, 60–63, 66–73, 75–77, 81
vitalism, 8, 38, 41

water-soluble salts (electrolytes), 3, 28, 29, 88, 98
weapon salve, 50
Western esotericism, 32
World Health Organization, 2
World War I, 113

yin/yang, 110

Zimpel, Friedrich, 87–89, 93
Zosimos of Panopolis, 16, 18

Therapeutic Index—Physical Symptoms

abdominal pain, 116
acidity, 124, 142, 143
addiction, 143
adrenal glands, 114
aging, 120, 121, 130, 149
alcohol, 3, 28, 30, 44, 67, 88, 89, 93, 97, 99, 102, 103, 106, 107, 129, 139, 161, 162
alcoholism, 117, 159
allergies, 124, 140, 158
Alzheimer's disease, 151
amputations, 114
analgesic, 110, 138, 162
anemia, 119, 158, 162, 163, 164
aneurism, 109
angina pectoris, 126
antibacterial, 109, 112, 113, 129, 146
antibiotic, 5, 152
antidepressant, 133, 138
antidote, 116, 117
antifungal, 113, 132
antihemorrhagic, 113
anti-inflammatory, 113, 138
antimicrobial, 109, 132
antiseptic, 110, 113, 129, 138, 148, 152
antispasm, 110, 148, 152, 155
antitumor, 115
antiviral, 113, 146
appendicitis, 119, 141
aspirin, 8, 9, 110
asthma, 1, 87, 98, 116, 119, 152, 154, 155, 156
astringent, 110, 139

babies, 113, 132
back, 10, 129
beautifier, 129, 132, 149, 154
bedwetting, 129
bile, 40, 114, 116, 132, 143
bladder, 127, 139, 142, 158, 159
bleeding, 109, 113, 129, 153, 155
blood, 25, 28, 40, 44, 55, 47, 58, 73, 94, 98, 109, 113, 114, 117, 135, 136, 149, 159, 162, 163, 164

bloodletting, 41, 44, 82
blood loss, 113, 114
blood pressure and hypertension, 109, 126, 127, 133, 148, 150, 153
blood sugar, 152, 162
blood vessels, 109, 127, 146, 155, 162
bones, 129, 130, 137, 159, 162, 163
brain, 25, 52, 59, 72, 146, 148, 149, 159, 151, 152, 153
breastfeeding, 111, 152
bronchitis, 154
bruises, 109, 138, 142
burns, 113, 115, 135, 136, 138, 148, 154

cancer, 1, 4, 38, 73, 114, 118, 121, 135, 149, 158, 166
Candida (thrush), 132
carminative, 110, 132, 133
catabolism, 142
catarrh, 133, 152
chest pain, 116, 126
chilliness, 85, 98, 114, 120, 149
chronic disease, 1, 4, 11, 84, 115, 117, 119, 121, 127, 135, 158
circulation, 4, 96, 97, 114, 146, 148, 150, 162
cleanser, 112, 116, 129, 135, 136, 154, 158, 160
clots, 109, 110
cold, 98, 114, 126, 149, 158, 163
colds, 85, 109, 145, 153, 154
conjunctivitis, 132
constipation, 119, 120, 158, 159
contractions, 111, 115
coronary thrombosis, 114
corpulence, 132
cough, 116, 119
cuts, 113, 115, 138
cystitis, 129, 135

delirium, 141
deodorant, 133
dermatitis 144
detox, 94, 98, 109, 110, 136, 137, 158, 161, 163
diabetes, 1, 4, 137, 142, 152, 158, 159, 162

diaper rash, 113
diarrhea, 119, 158
digestion, 5, 57, 97, 98, 99, 113, 132, 133, 140, 145, 146, 147, 148, 152, 154, 155, 158
diuretic, 9, 127, 129, 133, 135, 137, 143, 155, 158, 162
dropsy (water retention), 49, 119, 126, 135, 136, 141, 155, 159. See also edema
drugs, 2, 8, 9, 11, 68, 73, 86, 139, 140, 149, 159
dyspnea, 126, 154

eczema, 154, 156
edema, 119, 120, 137, 155. See also dropsy
elimination, 119, 121, 137, 162
emetic, 41, 82, 118, 155
energy deficit, 2, 4, 8
enteritis, 1
epilepsy, 134, 138, 150, 153
exhaustion, 98, 114, 143, 148
expectorant, 133, 139, 155
eyes, 19, 28, 49, 132, 137, 144, 154, 158

fatigue, 4, 117, 120, 130, 133, 148, 158
fever, 49, 85, 109, 110, 135, 145, 146
fingers, 138
flatulence, 98, 132, 152

galactogue, 115, 134
gallbladder, 114, 142, 158
gallstone colic, 116, 119
gargle, 113, 136
genitourinary system, 136
glands, 114, 135, 137, 142
glandular fever, 135
gout, 69, 130
grazes, 115
gunshot wounds, 113

hair, 129
headaches, 111, 116, 126, 130, 139, 140, 141, 142, 143, 145, 146, 148, 152, 158
heart, 1, 3, 97, 119, 126, 127, 128, 137, 145, 147, 148, 155
hernia, 141
herpes, 146
HIV, 115

hormones, 66, 136
hypertension. *See* blood pressure
hypochondria, 116, 119

immunity, 5, 12, 71, 72, 73, 74. 94, 119, 145, 158, 163
indigestion, 5, 132
infection, 4, 94, 123, 129, 146, 152
infertility, 110
inflammation, 83, 87, 135, 136, 152
influenza (flu), 1, 3, 145, 153, 154
injury, 12, 53, 110, 129, 138
insomnia, 117, 139, 154, 158
intestines, 98, 143, 152

jaundice, 119, 158
joints, 129, 130, 137, 149, 158

kidneys, 98, 125, 127, 130, 131, 136, 154, 155, 158, 159

leucorrhea, 119
liver, 25, 87, 116, 117, 118, 119, 121, 123, 132, 142, 143, 144, 157, 158, 160
lungs, 25, 153, 154, 156, 164
lymphatic system, 110, 113, 119, 121, 135, 136, 137

menopause, 129, 152
menorrhagia, 110
menstrual problems, 119, 122, 123, 149
metabolism, 3, 57, 119, 121, 135, 146, 149, 158, 163
metrorrhagia, 110, 116
middle age, 130
migraines, 142, 143, 148
mouth, 142, 152, 159
mouthwash, 113, 136, 140
muscles, 114, 132
mushroom poisoning, 117
myalgias, 4
myalgic encephalopathy (ME), 148

nails, 109, 129
nausea, 123, 160
neck, 133, 135, 137, 143

nerves, 72, 124, 134, 136, 137, 138, 139, 140, 143, 145, 146, 147, 149, 151, 152, 162, 163
nervous exhaustion, 139
nipples, 113
nosebleed, 108, 109, 113

obesity, 142, 159. *See also* corpulence
occupational disease, 43
operations, pre- and post-, 129

pain, 110, 119, 122, 126, 129, 130, 138, 139, 140, 141, 142, 149, 158, 159, 160, 162
  aching, 116
  burning, 135, 142
  chest, 118, 126
  chronic, 128
  dull, 129
  period pain, 109, 110
  rheumatic, 129, 149
  shooting, 138
  stomach, 119
  violent, 137
palpitations, 145
pancreas, 123, 142, 158
pathology, 4, 70, 71, 74, 84, 86, 159
periodicity, 142
pins and needles, 138
pneumonia, 1, 83, 85
poison, 22, 38, 41, 43, 53, 57, 68, 72, 117, 126, 153
postpartum, 113
potassium, 9, 97, 120, 123, 127, 133, 152, 155, 158, 159
potassium deficiency, 120
poultices, 142
pregnancy, 111, 115, 122, 123, 134, 150, 153, 164
premature aging, 120, 121, 149
prostate, 136, 162
psoriasis, 136, 154
pulse, 38, 49, 126, 148

radiation, 113
respiration, 52, 116, 133, 152, 153, 154, 155, 156

rheumatism, 4, 121, 129, 142, 149, 162

Salmonella enterica, 132
scalds, 135, 142
sciatica, 116
seasonal affective disorder (SAD), 114, 140
sedative, 126, 145, 146, 155
shock, 8, 12, 98
shortness of breath, 119, 126, 164
sickness, 125, 142
sides of the body
　　left, 119, 126
　　right, 129, 158
sinus, 142
skin, 111, 113, 114, 118, 123, 124, 132, 135,
　　136, 137, 140, 149, 154, 156, 158, 160,
　　162
sleep, 3, 117, 154, 158, 162
snakebite, 116, 135
spinal column, 130, 137
spleen, 25, 87, 116, 118, 119, 120, 121, 158,
　　159
Staphylococcus, 113, 152
Streptococcus, 113
stings, 115, 135, 138, 145, 161
stomach, 57, 94, 119, 132, 142, 147, 152
stones, 116, 127, 135
stroke, 1, 3, 109
styptic, 109, 110, 112, 113
sunburn, 154
suppuration, 113
surgery, 2, 98, 113, 140
sweating (perspiration), 41, 109, 117, 142,
　　143, 145, 152, 154, 158
syphilis, 43

teeth, 130, 157, 159
teething, 123
tendons, 114
tetanus, 138
thirst, 123, 149
throat, 5, 124, 135, 136, 142, 152, 153, 156
thrush, 132
thyroid, 142, 147
tonic, 110, 126, 135, 145, 151
tongue, 135, 136, 142

tonsils, 119, 135, 152
toothache, 109
tooth extraction, 113, 138
toxic, 3, 98, 110, 117, 126, 137, 154, 155,
　　159, 160, 161, 163
toxins, 110, 137, 161
trauma, 114, 155
tuberculosis, 1, 151

ulcers, 113, 135, 142, 152
urinary system, 129, 130, 135, 136, 137, 153,
　　154, 158, 162
uterus, 119, 136

veins, 113, 129, 136, 146
vascular system, 110, 148, 149
venereal disease, 118
vertigo, 111, 152
vision, 143, 158
vomiting, 116, 123

water retention. *See* dropsy, edema
weakness, 11, 53, 72, 94, 97, 100, 119, 120,
　　121, 126, 129, 130, 139, 140, 147, 148,
　　152, 163
wounds, 50, 72, 109, 110, 111, 112, 113,
　　114, 129, 138, 140, 142, 163

Therapeutic Index— Mental and Emotional Symptoms

absentminded, 117
aggression, 25, 75, 125, 128
ambition, 114, 120
anger, 12, 73, 110, 114, 117, 126, 128, 146,
　　159, 160
anxiety, 96, 114, 123, 139, 140, 144, 145,
　　146, 147, 151, 154, 156
apathy, 4, 12
assertiveness, 25, 114, 125, 164

compassion, 128
competitiveness, 114
confidence, 133, 150
concentration, 134, 148
courage, 12, 132, 133, 163, 164

delusions, 155
depression, 120, 133, 138, 139, 140, 143, 145, 150, 151, 159
despair, 12, 73, 127
despondency, 4, 114, 144
discipline, 118
dread, 114
dreams, 14, 41, 110, 143, 154, 155
drive, lack of, 120

empathy, 12, 94, 124, 125
endurance, 114, 118, 130, 133
existential fears, 110, 147

fastidious, 10, 120
fear, 43, 77, 114, 126, 130, 136, 139, 140, 146, 147, 155, 156
fright, 114, 154, 155
forgetful, 63, 117

grief, 12, 127, 128, 155

heroic medicine, 41, 82
heroism, 109, 114
humor, 120
hurried, 123, 124, 126

idealism, 120, 163
imagination, 43, 116, 139, 153
impatience, 123, 124, 126, 153
integrity, 118
intuition, 110
irritability, 4, 122, 124, 126, 130, 136, 159

jealousy, 12
joy, 73, 133, 160
Jupiter, 24, 25, 115, 118, 141, 144, 145, 157, 159

love, 65, 111, 128, 146, 155, 160

Mars, 111, 112, 114, 121, 124, 125, 128, 160, 163, 164
melancholy, 116, 117, 120, 133, 139, 147
memory, 134, 147, 148, 150, 151, 152, 153
mental-emotional, 2, 65, 94, 119, 133, 134, 143, 148, 150, 151, 154, 159

Mercury, 121, 124, 125, 127, 133, 139, 145, 147, 151, 153, 156
moon, 44, 110, 145, 147, 150, 151, 153
moralizing, 118, 120

nervous, 72, 124, 134, 136, 138, 139, 140, 143, 145, 146, 147, 151, 152, 162, 163
nightmares, 117, 129

oversensitive, 122
overwork, 143

pessimism, 19, 121, 148
poise, 121
protection from outside influences, 133

reasoning, 124, 125, 152, 153
relationship problems, 140, 143
resentment, 96, 110
responsibility, 120, 130
rigidity, 120, 130, 137

Saturn, 118, 121, 128, 130, 134, 137
sedative, 126, 145, 146, 155
self-expression, 125, 139
sensitive, 11, 122, 139, 140, 144, 153, 158
sorrow, 127, 128
spiritual aspiration, 124, 128, 130, 142, 144, 146, 150, 151, 152
stress, 4, 5, 73, 94, 123, 136, 139, 143, 145, 146, 148, 162
sun, 30, 114, 125, 127, 128, 137, 140
sunburn, 154

tears, 120, 143
temper, 123

Venus, 25, 111, 128, 134, 136
vision (sight), 143
visions, 110, 111, 155
vulnerability, 110

will, 64, 65, 66, 130, 139, 140, 147, 148, 163
work, 132, 143, 159